MEAL PREP COOKBOOK FOR MEN

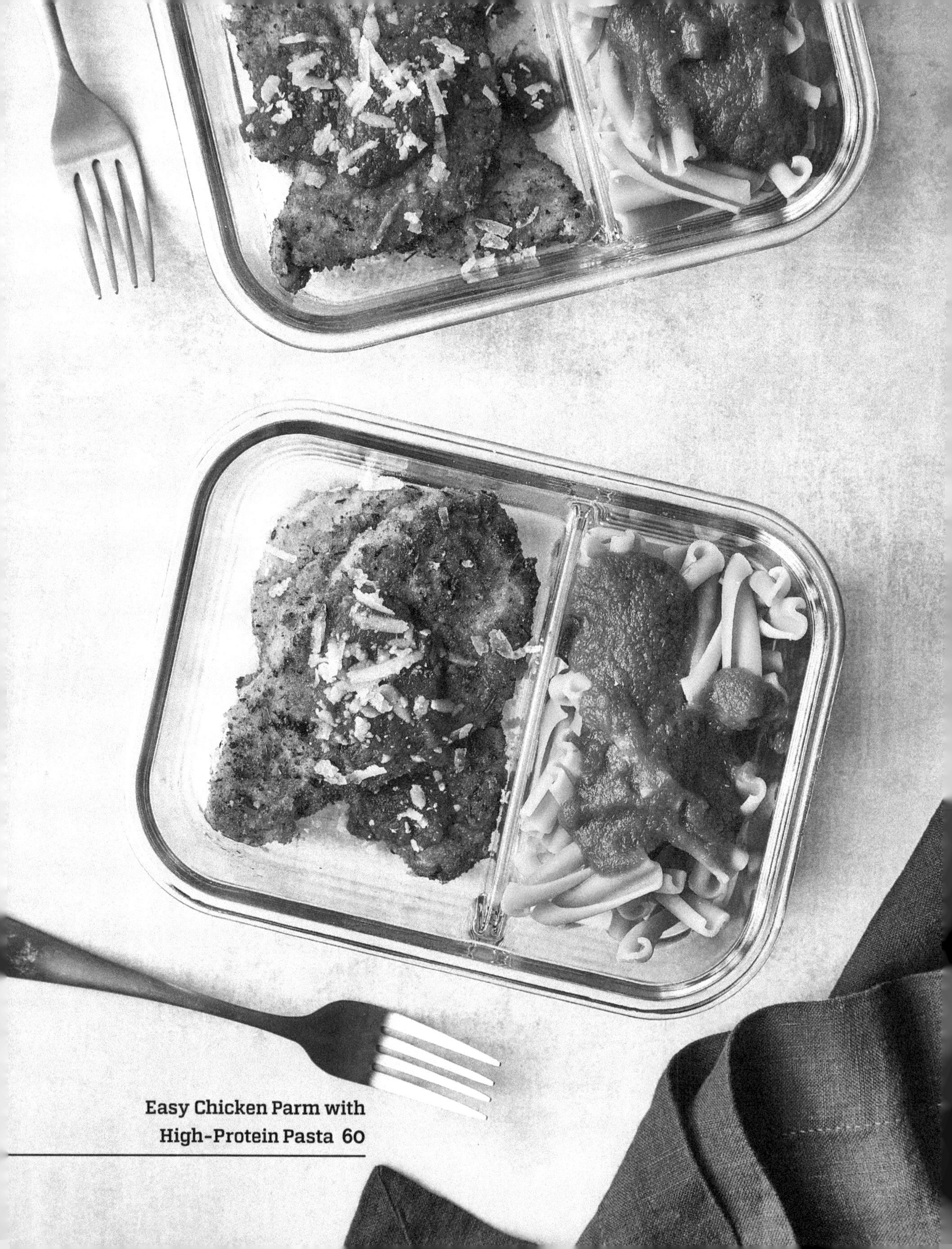

Easy Chicken Parm with High-Protein Pasta 60

MEAL PREP COOKBOOK FOR MEN

FUEL YOUR FITNESS WITH HEALTHY MEALS

TED KALLMYER, M.Ed.

PHOTOGRAPHY BY HÉLÈNE DUJARDIN

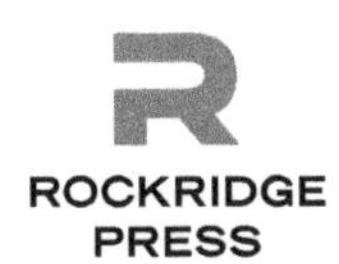

Interior and Cover Designer: Eric Pratt
Art Producer: Tom Hood
Editor: Anna Pulley
Production Editor: Mia Moran
Production Manager: Jose Olivera

Paperback ISBN: 978-1-64876-292-5 | eBook ISBN: 978-1-64876-293-2

R0

I dedicate this book to the thousands of nutritional coaching clients I've had over the years. Their success and transformation is the inspiration that keeps me going.

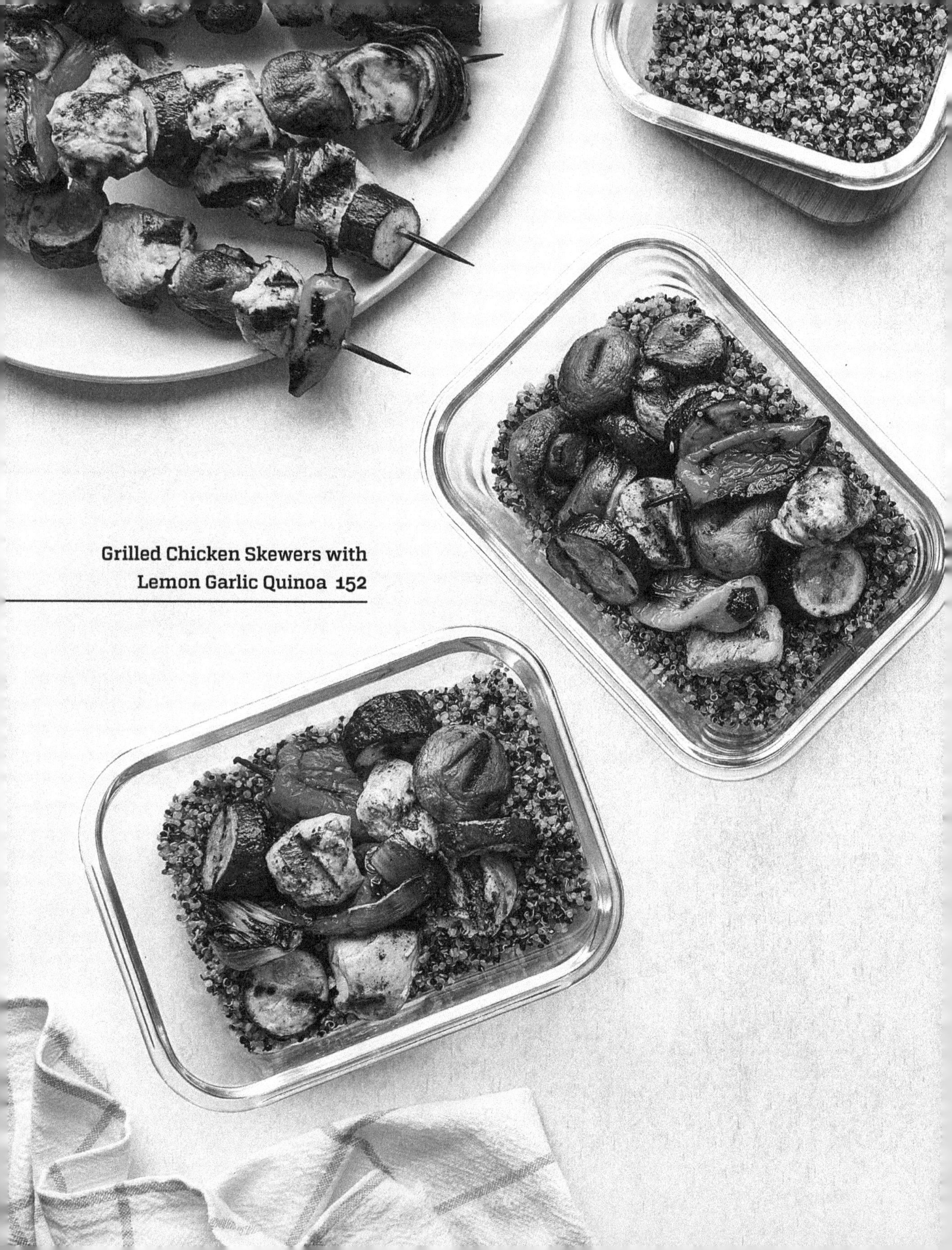

Grilled Chicken Skewers with Lemon Garlic Quinoa 152

CONTENTS

Introduction

Congratulations on deciding to make positive changes to your diet to fuel your workouts! Whether you're a beginner or a seasoned athlete, this book will help ensure you give your body the materials for success in achieving increased fitness and vitality.

I've always been interested in looking and feeling fit. However, I had no idea how to eat in order to achieve this. In my high school years, I thought skipping lunch would get me there. In my 20s, I thought SlimFast and ab belts were the way to go. It wasn't until my late 30s that I finally understood proper nutrition was key. I was so blown away by my personal transformation that I began blogging about it. Eventually, I became certified in fitness nutrition and developed nutritional programs to help others make sense of this confusing topic. I've now been a nutritional coach and the author behind HealthyEater.com for about 10 years.

The number one thing I try to instill in my clients—besides carbs not being the devil—is that if you want to be fit and athletic, your diet matters. Your body is a complex machine, so it makes sense to give that machine the right type and amount of fuel if you want it to go the distance. What you eat before a workout and what you eat after makes a big difference in how far you can go and how fast you'll get there.

Meal prep is a powerful tool to help you do just that because it accomplishes two main purposes. First, it shows you what balanced nutrition looks like for your desired goals. Second, it acknowledges one of the biggest obstacles people have when they want to change their diet: *time*. Many people have good intentions to eat better, but work, family, and social functions quickly thwart those good intentions. Who has time to cook healthy dinners or pack healthy lunches every day? Meal prep ensures that you always have healthy meals ready to eat.

This book has an easy-to-follow format so you can begin eating better quickly. First, I'll discuss nutrition and clear up some myths surrounding the topic. I'll break down how to eat if you want to lose weight and/or gain lean muscle. Next, I'll show you that cooking doesn't have to be complicated and doesn't require a lot of expensive equipment. I'll follow up with tips for cooking success. Then, you'll find six meal prep plans to follow, depending on your unique fitness needs complete with delicious recipes that store easily and well. Plus, I'll give you 42 more recipes for designing your own weekly meal prep plans. None are complicated, require fancy ingredients, or take ages to cook. Many are just healthier versions of classics, designed to be super simple and super tasty.

No matter where you're starting from, this fitness meal prep cookbook will help you get to the next level and keep you properly nourished on the way.

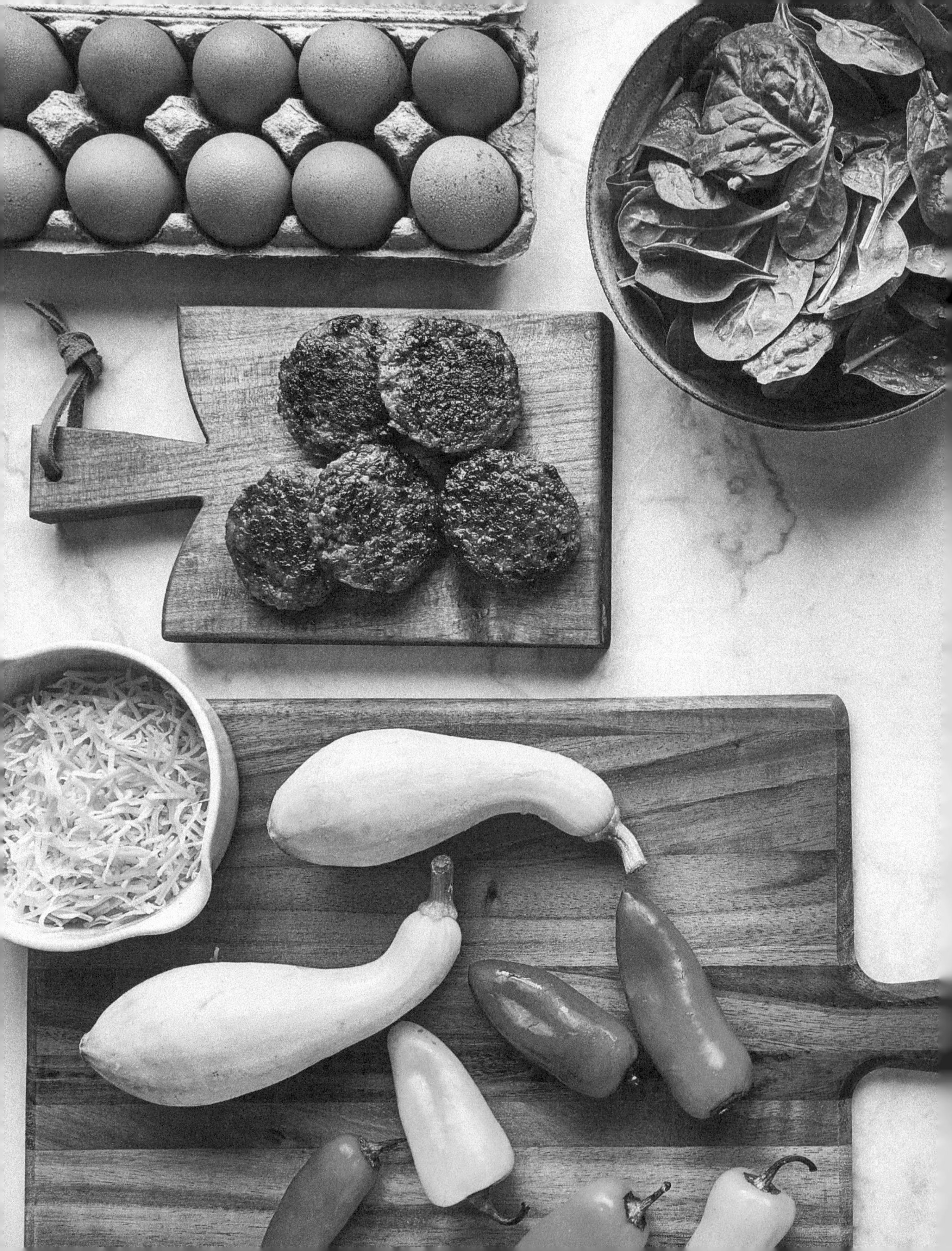

PART ONE

THE FOOD AND FITNESS CONNECTION

Throughout this book you'll see me refer to your body as a machine, and it's important you start thinking that way. Your body needs energy to operate, and food is how it gets that energy. In high school, I thought skipping lunch would give me the physique I wanted, and at the same time, I signed up to run long-distance in track. I doubt I need to spell out what happened. I crashed and burned big-time. I couldn't keep up, and I developed an overuse injury. I wasn't giving my machine enough energy to thrive, and it let me know.

In part 1, I'll give you the knowledge my high-school self didn't have: what the right nutrition is, how it should match up with your fitness type, and how to prepare the right meals that will fuel your machine.

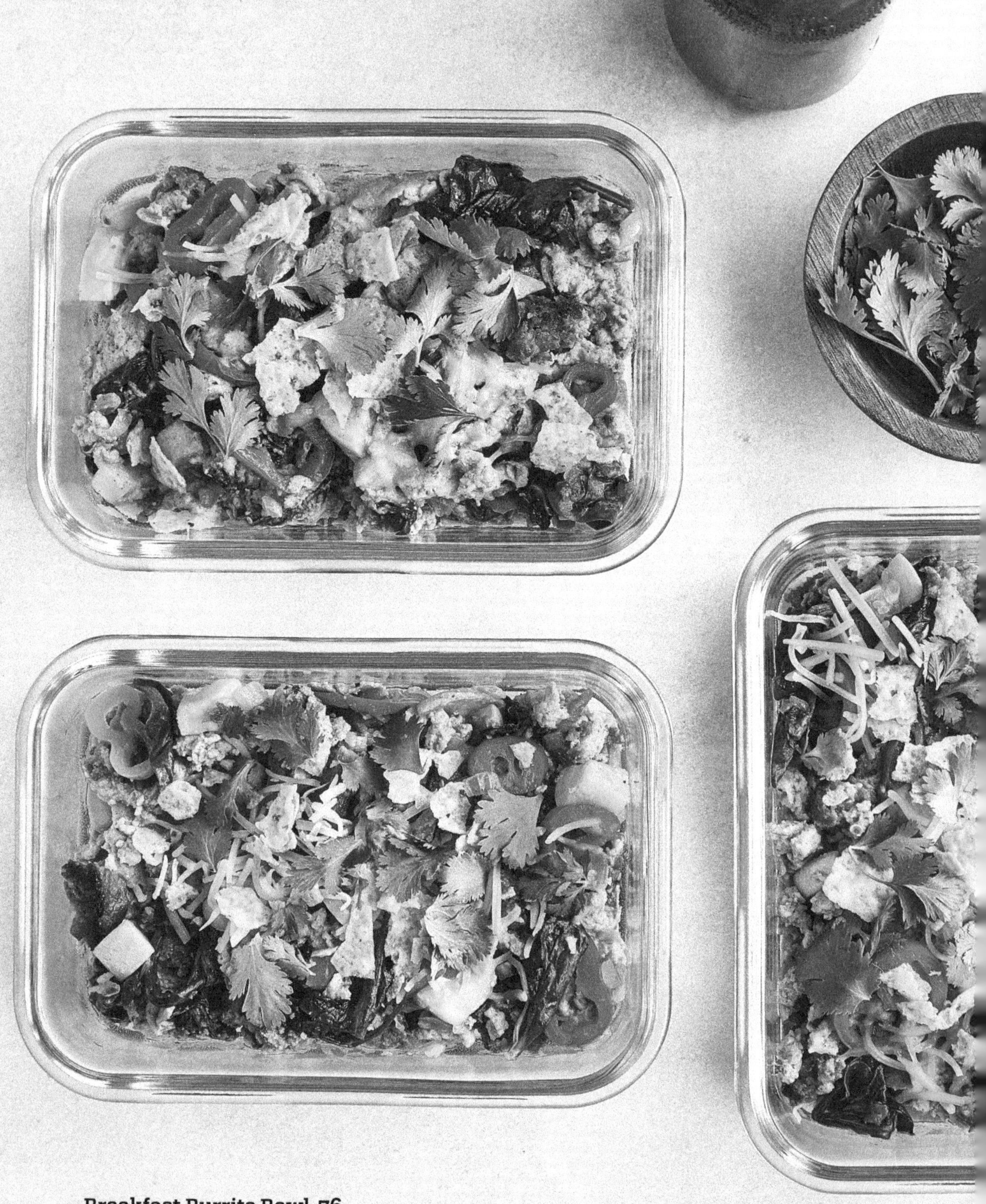

Breakfast Burrito Bowl 76

CHAPTER ONE

PREPPING FOR SUCCESS

Education is powerful, so here's your crash course in nutrition to prime you for success no matter what your fitness goals may be. We'll discuss basic nutrition, weed out pervasive myths, and curate your kitchen for easy meal prep.

Eating Right for Your Body and Activity Level

Humans come in all shapes and sizes and therefore shouldn't all be eating the same thing. Many factors go into finding the right eating plan, like age, sex, height, weight, and activity level. I created the recipes in this book with this in mind so they can easily be adapted to your specific needs. Although these recipes are great for all people who enjoy fitness, men and women often have different nutritional needs. This primarily has to do with the fact that men on average have more muscle mass, which requires more energy to maintain. Most men have a higher basal metabolic rate and therefore need more daily protein.

If you're thinking, "sounds complicated," don't worry; meal prep removes most of the guesswork and ensures you get the appropriate amount of energy and macronutrients for your unique body and activity level.

Defining Macros and Micros

Your body obtains energy and raw materials from three types of macronutrients: carbohydrates, protein, and fat.

Carbohydrates—Carbs are the main and preferred energy source for your body. They're further broken down into starches, sugars, and fiber. Starches are complex carbohydrates and take longer to digest, whereas sugars are simple carbohydrates and are digested fairly quickly. Fiber is mostly indigestible but essential for gut health.

Protein—Protein is used for growth, repair, and other vital processes. Proteins are made of amino acids combined in different ways depending on bodily need. You only need a finite amount per day; if you eat more, it's converted to energy.

Fats—Fat is needed for healthy brain and nervous tissue, hormone production, healthy blood, and much more. Fats are classified as saturated, monounsaturated, and polyunsaturated. Too much of the wrong kinds of fat can cause excess cholesterol production, which can result in cardiovascular problems. A good rule is to get most of your fat from plants, which contain predominately unsaturated fat.

Your body also needs micronutrients—minerals, vitamins, antioxidants, and electrolytes. An easy way to get the necessary micronutrients is to eat a lot of whole foods, predominately from plants, which are micronutrient powerhouses.

Sodium, a main component of salt, is a micronutrient. It's easy to consume too much because sodium is in so many food products. A whole foods-based diet gives you more control because you add salt yourself. Typically, if you have healthy blood pressure and don't exercise too much, limit sodium to less than 2,300 mg per day. However, if you're active and sweat a lot, your intake can be much greater. On really active days, keep your daily intake under 4,000 mg.

All the recipes in this book have a balanced set of macros, use whole-food ingredients, and deliver loads of vegetables to ensure excellent overall nutrition.

CALCULATING YOUR DAILY MACROS

Because your energy needs are based on your unique stats, goals, and activity level, it's important to calculate how much of each macro is appropriate for you. One of the most respected formulas for men is the Mifflin-St. Jeor formula that estimates **Resting Energy Expenditure (REE)**:

$$10 \times \text{weight (kg)} + 6.25 \times \text{height (cm)} - 5 \times \text{age (y)} + 5 = \text{REE}$$

Because most people don't just lie in bed all day, we factor in an activity factor of 1.2 to account for general movement.

Your REE × 1.2 = your sedentary Total Daily Energy Expenditure (TDEE)

This calculates your energy needs on a day you don't exercise. If you do plan to exercise, estimate how many calories you burn during your workouts and add that to your sedentary TDEE. This allows you to factor in your energy needs when you exercise. From there, to calculate your macros, you establish a healthy ratio (40% carbs, 30% protein, and 30% fat is suitable for most active people). Multiply your TDEE and each percentage. Then divide both carbs and protein by 4 and fat by 9 to calculate how many grams of each macro to eat. If that seems like a lot of math, don't stress. Online calculators can do it for you—one of the best is my own (see Resources, page 168).

In creating the meal preps for this book, I used an average-height male (5'9") weighing 175 pounds as a point of reference. You may need to adjust the portions depending on your unique needs and goals.

How to Eat Like an Athlete

Professional athletes eat big. Athletes understand their body is a machine and energy is required to make the mechanisms operate correctly. When swimmer Michael Phelps was competing in the Olympics, he ate 8,000 to 10,000 calories daily to maintain his weight and training schedule.

Your diet has to match the level of athleticism you're aspiring to. You need to understand how much energy your body requires at rest and how much more it needs when training.

Knowing your TDEE and the right balance of macronutrients to resupply what your body is using is paramount. If you're a bodybuilder, focus on higher protein and moderate carbs. More amino acids will be needed to rebuild the muscle broken down during your lifting sessions. If you're a runner, focus on higher carbs and moderate protein. Your muscles need plenty of fuel for those runs and to replace spent glycogen stores.

It's been proven that processed foods containing refined carbs and unhealthy fats increase your risk of heart disease, cancer, and early death. What hasn't been as well researched is how such foods affect your mood, energy levels, and overall feelings of well-being. An athletic physique is great, but if you feel like crap, what's the point?

I believe a holistic approach to diet and nutrition is crucial for optimal health in body, mind, and spirit. A diet rich in vegetables, fruit, whole grains, and high-quality proteins not only supplies the energy you need immediately but also delivers the micronutrients to thrive, fight disease, and live a long, healthy life. It's like putting ultra-premium in your engine instead of regular unleaded gas.

Here are more specific guidelines whether you're focused on strength training, cardio, or both.

Eating for Cardio

Cardio activities quickly use up your body's available glucose and glycogen. How fast this can be compensated for and replaced depends on how you eat before and afterward.

Eating carbs before and after a cardio workout replenishes spent glycogen stores in your muscles. For long-duration cardio, it's important to fuel during the session as well. Long-distance runners are always refueling to avoid the dreaded "bonk," when energy gets so low you can't think straight and eventually have to stop.

If you're training for a marathon, it's important to eat properly for several weeks before the event, otherwise you could wreak havoc on your digestive system. Running a race with stomach cramps will quickly do a person in, and bathrooms aren't always available.

Eating for Strength Training

People who lift weights need a good supply of carbs to fuel their workouts, and also adequate protein. The goal of weight training is to break down the muscle group you're working on and rebuild it stronger. Therefore, your diet should have higher levels of protein to give your muscles the materials for repair and growth.

One myth is that you should eat 1 gram of protein per pound of body weight. That isn't accurate. Your protein needs should relate to your lean mass rather than your total body weight, especially if you have a few pounds of excess fat to lose. Unused protein is converted to energy, and because carbs (an efficient energy source) are readily available and less costly, eating excess protein is throwing money down the drain.

For strength training, eat some carbs beforehand and a protein-rich meal or snack within 30 minutes afterward. If your workout was 45 to 60 minutes long, 30 to 50 grams of protein is recommended.

Bodybuilding or Developing Lean Muscle

There are two basic approaches to gaining muscle.

Bulking—Eat a lot of food and gain muscle as well as fat.

Lean gains—Eat slightly more than the energy requirements of your body to gain muscle but not gain fat.

Which is best? In my opinion, the lean gains method is the way to go. Gaining and then losing fat is hard on the body and doesn't make economic sense.

Eating for Cardio and Strength

Many people enjoy exercise that's a combination of cardio and strength. Cross-training works out your heart and strengthens your muscles, although it's a little less focused than a dedicated weight-lifting program. Eating for cardio and strength requires slightly higher protein than strictly cardio activity and slightly higher carbs than strictly strength training. You have to fuel your workouts and also provide your muscles with the raw materials they need.

For this type of training, follow the rule for strength training. Have some carbs beforehand and a protein-rich meal or snack within 30 minutes afterward. Shoot for 20 to 40 grams of protein if your workout was 45 to 60 minutes long.

For cross-training competitors engaging in events that last a good portion of the day, fuel before and after each event, but keep it light and focus on easy-to-digest foods. It's helpful to plan your snacks and even eat them leading up to your event.

The Role of Water

Your body is about 60 percent water, and almost every bodily process depends on it. However, your body conserves and recycles water, so you don't need to replace it all daily. Under normal conditions (absent high temperatures and intense exercise), you need about 64 fluid ounces daily. This is water from all sources, including what you drink and eat. (Keep in mind that alcohol dehydrates, so for every alcoholic drink, drink a glass of plain water.)

If it's hot and you're sweating a lot, you need more water. If you're working out intensely, you need more water. In extreme conditions, 84 to 100 fluid ounces is recommended, depending on how much you sweat and how much you weigh. Some of that water should contain electrolytes to replace minerals lost in sweat. Electrolytes are needed for nervous tissue function, so your muscles fire as they should, and are vital for health and athletic performance. But think twice before you reach for that sports drink: Many are loaded with sugar and artificial colors and flavors. If you sweat profusely during exercise, get some electrolyte packets or concentrates. They're cost effective and come in all-natural, low-sugar, and sugar-free brands.

Being hydrated helps you feel energetic, alert, full, and at your best. Have a drink every hour or more frequently if exercising. Thirst is a good signal that it's time for a drink.

How Can I Lose Weight?

Even for athletic individuals, it's common to carry around a few extra pounds of fat. Unfortunately, it's a common misunderstanding that active men can eat as much they want because they work out. I've got news for you: Never rely on exercise to keep you from gaining weight. Adjust your diet first and then use exercise to allow you to eat a little more.

To lose weight, you need to eat fewer calories than your body requires to maintain itself, but not too many fewer. It's important to find a balance that allows fat loss but doesn't sacrifice the muscle tissue that you're working hard to build or maintain. Remember the TDEE calculation? For safe weight loss of about one pound per week, deduct 20 percent from your sedentary TDEE and your exercise-adjusted TDEE. Anything more risks muscle tissue loss, which eventually lowers your metabolic rate. Slow and steady is best. Those who go for fast and furious end up gaining the weight back quickly once they resume their old eating habits.

Meal prep is a great way to ensure that you reduce calories properly and always have the right amount of food. You simply eat the preportioned meals that deliver the right amount of energy for gradual weight loss.

If you need help holding yourself accountable, hire a professional to do your calculations, keep you motivated, and encourage you when you feel like giving up. There's no shame in asking for help, especially when your health and longevity are concerned.

Tune In to What Your Body Is Saying

Just like any machine, your body needs regular maintenance and care. Listen to the signals. Pain or fatigue are signals to slow down and take a rest. It's okay if you can't work out as hard as the person next to you; everyone is different and at different stages in their fitness journeys. When engaging in new activities, start at a comfortable pace and gradually increase. If you go in guns blazing, you'll probably regret it. You may even get injured, which derails progress. Take a rest day when your body is fatigued. Get plenty of sleep and be in tune with what your body is telling you. You're in charge.

Healthy Can Be Delicious

Many people think healthy eating is boring, bland, and filled with nothing but broccoli and dry chicken. This couldn't be further from the truth. In this book, you'll find healthier versions of classics and new recipes that are all full of flavor. As mentioned, the most important aspect of eating healthy is eating a whole-food diet rich in plant-based foods. Seasonings, spices, and even healthy fat are good. I want to emphasize that your diet doesn't have to be perfect to be healthy. If you practice healthy eating habits 80 to 85 percent of the time, you'll be in great shape.

WHAT ABOUT CHEAT DAYS?

"Cheat day" implies you're doing something bad or forbidden, so let's use "free days" instead. Being diligent 80 to 85 percent of the time will help you reach your goals. It's okay to relax a little from time to time, have an indulgent meal, and enjoy life's special moments. One common incorrect assumption is that people need to starve themselves the day after a free day—but that isn't healthy. Rather than starving yourself, return to your regular eating plan. Be smart and monitor how many free days you allow yourself, as that will affect the time it takes to achieve your fitness goals, especially if one of those goals is weight loss. One day per week or one day biweekly is usually a good goal. Keep free days within reason, but don't be afraid to have some.

Where Does My Activity Fit In?

Is your fitness training cardio, strength, or a combination of both? Whereas running is obviously cardio and weight lifting is obviously strength, some activities might not be as clear. This table should help you determine where your exercise of choice fits in.

CARDIO	STRENGTH	CARDIO/STRENGTH
Aerobic classes, basketball, cross-country skiing, cycling, dance, ellipticals, fast walking, hiking, in-line skating, pickleball, running, soccer, spinning, stairs/ stair machine, surfing, swimming, tennis	Body-weight exercises (push-ups, pull-ups, etc.), circuit training with weight machines, dead lifts, power lifting, TRX, weight lifting	CrossFit and other cross-training programs, HIIT workouts with weights, kickboxing, martial arts, Orange Theory, rock climbing, rowing, yoga

Celebrating Victories

Modern society tempts us to eat unhealthily. Making the decision to get fit and healthy is a huge accomplishment in itself. You're doing something most people don't do, so celebrate that. As you continue your fitness journey, list some realistic goals and celebrate each milestone, whether it's running two miles, losing five pounds, or eating healthy for two weeks. Celebrate and don't stop there. If your goal is to run a half-marathon, don't stop running once the event is over. And if you fail, don't let that stop you, either. Have some patience and extend grace to yourself.

LET THEM EAT SNACKS

Being overly hungry can lead to poor eating decisions, so plan some healthy snacks for the week and have them handy. Before a workout, a carb-rich snack is good. My go-to is fresh fruit. Bananas, apples, and mandarin oranges provide a healthy dose of carbs and also vitamins and minerals. After a workout, especially weight-bearing activity, have a protein-rich snack. Protein smoothies/shakes are good, as is uncured, low-sodium jerky. I've lifted weights for so many years I can barely stand the taste of a protein shake, so I have a can of tuna mixed with mayonnaise and crackers as my post-workout snack. I've included some pre- and post-workout snack recipes in this book so you'll have plenty of options.

Setting Up Your Healthy Kitchen

Whether you're new to cooking or a seasoned chef, having the right equipment, tools, and terminology is important. I remember making a grilled cheese with my iron in college, so my goal is to help you avoid similar catastrophes by preparing you to make the recipes in this book.

BRUSHING UP ON THE BASICS

As you dig into the recipes, some cooking terms may be unfamiliar. Don't stress; all the recipes are designed to be simple to make, with minimal steps involved, so here I'll cover the basics.

Bake—cook in the oven with the oven setting on bake and preheated to the given temperature

Beat—stir vigorously until the ingredients are uniformly combined

Chop—cut the food into smaller pieces of varied sizes

Dice—cut the food into small pieces or squares

Fillet—cut a piece of meat into a thin slice (e.g., to fillet a chicken breast, halve it horizontally, producing two thin fillets)

Sauté—soften in a little oil, usually over medium heat and stirred frequently

Simmer—let something cook at just under a boil or a very slow boil, so only an occasional bubble rises

Most recipes are pretty forgiving if you don't do things exactly right. Taste is the most important thing, so always choose taste over presentation.

Pantry MVPs

There are a few items to always keep stocked in your pantry, refrigerator, or freezer.

Albacore tuna, canned—a protein powerhouse and a quick way to get high-quality protein

Baking powder—used as a leavening agent to make things fluffy

Bananas—great pre-workout snacks; frozen ripe bananas are terrific for smoothies

Black beans—a staple of many vegetarian recipes, this flavorful legume is a great protein and carb source

Chickpea pasta—a higher-protein and lower-carb option than regular pasta

Chickpeas—a mild-flavored legume rich in protein and good carbs

Eggs—used in a multitude of recipes

Egg whites—provide a protein boost but without the fat and cholesterol of whole eggs

Frozen blueberries—a nutritional boost for smoothies, oatmeal, and desserts

Frozen mixed vegetables—a quick way to make stir-fries or add a healthy side dish

Milk or dairy-free alternative—adds richness to smoothies, sauces, and baked goods

Organic pasta sauce—a faster but still healthy alternative to homemade

Peanut and/or almond butter—both deliver a quick, satisfying snack containing all three macros

Tomatoes, diced and crushed, canned—from salsa to sauces, lycopene-rich canned tomatoes are essential

Whole wheat flour—essential for many dishes; gluten-free flour is fine, too

Keep It Spicy

Spices are "free" foods in that they add flavor but not calories. Here are five used frequently in the recipes in this book.

Black pepper—adds a little kick

Cinnamon—provides a complex flavor boost in savory and sweet dishes

Garlic powder—adds flavor and micronutrients

Oregano—boosts flavor

Sea salt—adds flavor and minerals and is healthier than refined table salt

Prepared sauces are another way to add flavor but not many calories. They speed up meal prep and make meals more interesting.

Hot sauce—the basis of "Buffalo sauce"; adds heat and tanginess

Reduced-sodium soy sauce—used in many Asian-inspired recipes

Teriyaki sauce—adds umami to stir-fries, rice bowls, and more

There are many different sauces and seasonings, so don't be afraid to experiment. There's no reason to ever eat dry, bland grilled chicken or plain vegetables.

Kitchen Power Tools

A few dishes, utensils, and appliances will make preparing the recipes in this book much easier.

Blender or **food processor**—a must-have for smoothies and great for other mixing/chopping tasks

Can opener—safe-edge can openers are best; they cut the seal, not the metal

Casserole dish—glass or nonstick metal

Cast-iron skillet—can be used on the stove top or in the oven. Buy one that's preseasoned. Never put cast iron in the dishwasher or use soap on it. To clean, use water and a scrubber sponge, dry on the stove, and coat with oil for storage.

Cutting boards—one for meats and one for vegetables. I keep a wooden one for vegetables and a plastic dishwasher-safe one for meats.

High-quality knives—you don't have to spend a lot on knives, but you do have to keep them sharp. Buy a quick sharpener along with your knife set.

Measuring cup and spoons—a must for new cooks, especially if you're tracking your macros

Mixing bowls—large, medium, and small

Nonstick skillet—for sautéing vegetables or panfrying meat with little to no oil. To keep nonstick pans in good shape, never heat them beyond medium and never use metal utensils

Pots—a good stainless steel set (2- to 5-quart, with lids)

Sheet pan—for roasting vegetables and meats. The big rectangular ones are the most versatile. Line with parchment paper for swift and easy cleanup.

Spatula—for stir-fries to scrambled eggs and much more

Tongs—to keep your hands safe when turning meat or serving hot food

Extra Gadgets

These items can make your chef life easier but aren't essential.

Electric hand mixer—can be used with mixing bowls, so simpler than a blender

Parchment paper—for lining baking sheets and dishes for easy cleanup

Slow cooker—things can cook while you get on with other things

Vegetable chopper—makes chopping/dicing onions, peppers, squash, and other vegetables a breeze

Once your kitchen is ready to go, you can start focusing on how to cook "the meal prep way." It's a bit different than traditional cooking, because all the recipes are designed to be stored, then reheated and eaten at a later date. The next chapter gives you the tools to be an expert meal prepper and take your fitness to new levels by preparing healthy meals.

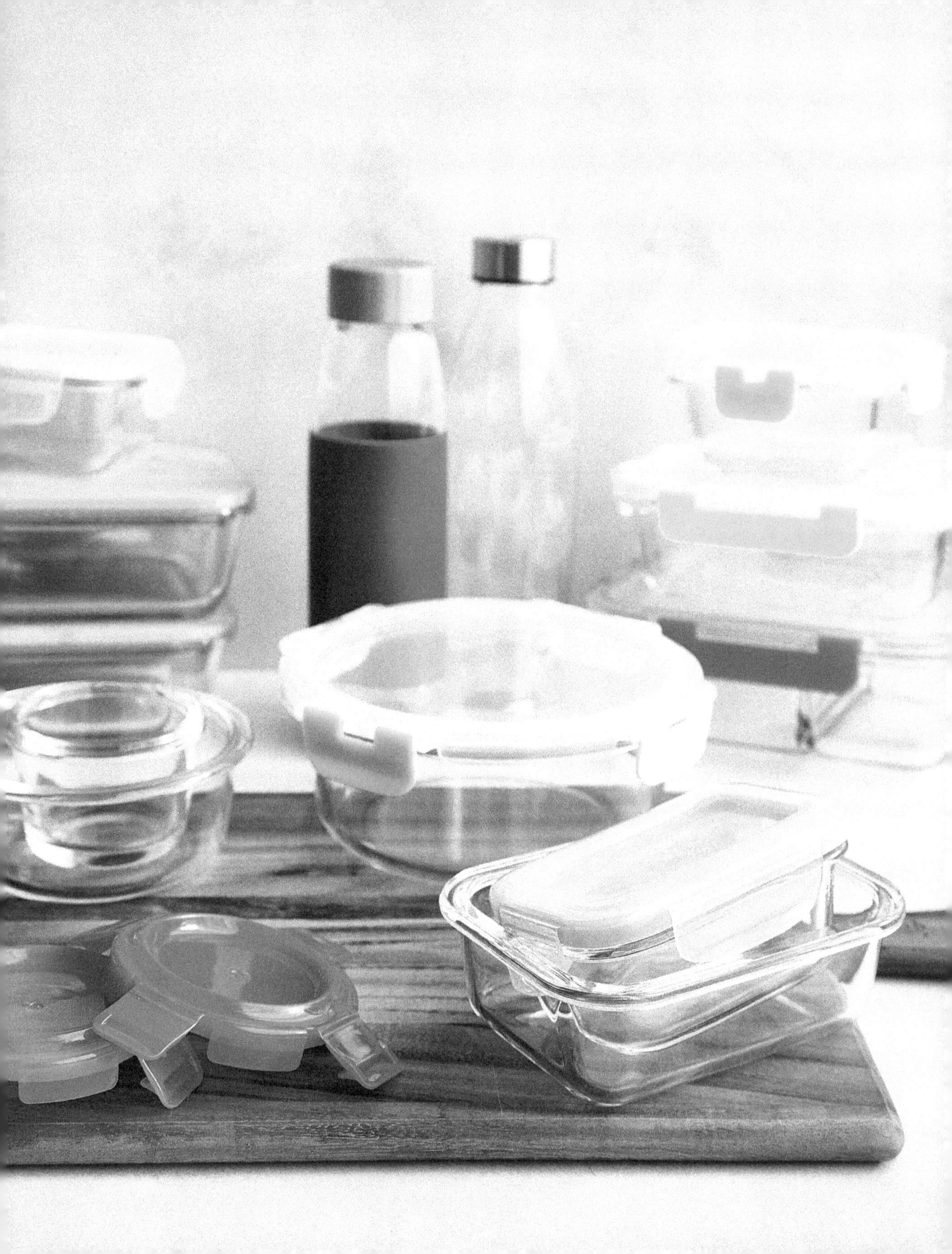

CHAPTER TWO

ALL ABOUT MEAL PREP

This is where I get into the meat and potatoes (no pun intended) of successful weekly meal prepping. I'll take you through each step and give you tips on bulk cooking, finding the right storage containers, and reheating things right so your meals taste as good as the day you made them.

Meal Prep for Fitness

The ultimate goal of meal prepping is to save you time and ensure that you give your body the nutrition it needs to accomplish your fitness goals, no matter how busy your schedule. Lack of time to cook is perhaps the number one excuse my clients make when it comes to eating better. So, let's nip that excuse in the bud, right now. Here are some reasons meal prep can transform your eating and thus transform your body/fitness level.

Time management—You'll only be devoting about four hours of one day to create a week's worth of meals, so no more stress about having to cook a healthy meal, finding a healthy lunch, or making time for a decent breakfast. All your meals for the week will be in the refrigerator or freezer.

Calorie/macro tracking—Your meals will be portioned according to your calorie and macro needs, so you'll know you're eating the correct amounts. You won't have to track what you're eating, stress over daily macro balance, or guess what you should be eating.

Consistency—One of the keys to achieving weight loss and fitness goals is consistency. Meal prep helps you be consistent by maintaining a calorie deficit (for weight loss) or maintaining a small calorie surplus (to gain lean muscle).

Hunger management—Meal prep helps you manage your hunger by always having filling meals and snacks on hand. A big impediment to success is becoming too busy to eat, thus becoming too hungry and therefore making bad food choices.

Cost effectiveness—Have you ever tracked how much money you spend eating out each month? Because all my recipes are healthy and economical, you'll probably save a significant amount of money.

Less food waste—About 50 percent of food in the United States gets thrown out. Meal prep means you use the entire recipe over the course of a week, so you'll no longer throw out leftovers or forget about something in the refrigerator. Meal prep uses the same ingredients in multiple meals, so ingredients won't go to waste.

At first glance, preparing a week's worth of meals may seem intimidating, but I assure you that it won't just save you time, it will make your busy week way less stressful.

Six-Step Prep

These six steps will help you become an expert meal prepper. As with anything new, there's a learning curve, so be patient with yourself and the process as you learn and find out what works best for you.

1. **Choose your prep day(s)—**Most meal preppers prep their meals on the weekend so that they'll be ready for the busy week ahead. The prep day is very flexible, so choose what works best for your schedule. If your days off are during the week, then meal prep on one of those days. You'll need to shop and cook, so plan to set aside four to six hours.
2. **Make your plan—**Decide which meal prep plan makes the most sense for the upcoming week. Consider what you'll be doing fitness-wise, then choose accordingly.
3. **Go shopping—**Each meal prep plan has a grocery list. You can refine the list by assessing what you already have in stock, then buy all the ingredients you'll need for the week's meals. If you hate going to the store, technology is at your fingertips. You can plug your list into the store's app or website, and they'll do all the shopping. They'll either bring your groceries out to your car or deliver them to your door.
4. **Prepare and cook—**When you begin, you may want to focus on one recipe at a time, so it'll take you a bit longer to meal prep. However, the more often you prep, the better you'll get at it, and you'll soon have multiple recipes cooking simultaneously. This is when a well-stocked kitchen comes in handy—you'll be using several pans and pots. A slow cooker can really help, since it's a more hands-off way to cook. Cooking can be fun, but cleanup can be dreaded. Using parchment paper on any pan that goes in the oven will make cleanup a snap.
5. **Portion and pack—**After a recipe is cooked, you'll want to divide the recipe between containers. All hot recipes will need to cool for about 15 minutes before portioning into containers. Bacteria can start growing at around 160°F, so you'll want to then put the containers in the refrigerator or freezer. If the dish will be eaten within the next five days, usually the refrigerator is fine. If not, put those portions in the freezer. If you don't have access to a

refrigerator at work, freezing your workday meals is a good idea since they will gradually thaw during the morning but remain safe.

6. **Grab and go—**Here comes the easy part. Each morning, eat your prepped breakfast at home (or at your desk when you get to work). Pack what you need for your workday (including pre- and post-workout snacks if you work out before returning home). Dinner will be waiting in the refrigerator.

Storage Is Key

Proper storage in the right kind of containers is important in meal prep. You don't want to be that guy who leaks sauce in the break room refrigerator. If you're following the meal preps in this book, prepping food once a week for five days' worth of meals/snacks, you'll need about 20 containers per week.

Choosing Your Containers

Luckily meal prep isn't new, so there are whole brands focused on this concept. The main things you want to consider is that the containers have an airtight and watertight seal, they're dishwasher- and microwave-safe, and they're infinite use. (Why put more litter in the landfill if we don't need to?) Crest, Bayco, Rubbermaid, and Fullstar are good brands and are available online. Rubbermaid is also found in most big box stores. Here are some notes on container types.

Glass—My favorite, because glass has infinite uses, doesn't stain or absorb odors, and is environmentally friendly. These are more expensive up front, but you don't need to replace them as often as plastic containers.

Plastic—More affordable, but with a few caveats. The plastic must be BPA-free and durable. Thinner plastic containers will wear out pretty quickly and end up in the garbage. Plastic can get stained and absorb odors.

Single and multicompartment—A mix of container types is handy as some meals will be "one pot" type meals whereas others can have a main and sides.

Stackable/nestable—Useful, especially if you don't have a lot of storage space.

Takeout containers—You may have a stack of these already. As long as they still seal and are uncracked, feel free to use them until you can invest in glass containers.

Keep It Going

As the weeks go by, you'll develop your own process and time-savers. Here are a few that will help you right out of the gate. Remember that your overall goal is to eat better so you can stay on track with your fitness plan and meet your goals. The more efficient and streamlined the meal prep process, the better.

Cook in batches—Cooking multiple meals at the same time is the most time-efficient option. Some recipes can be doubled, and extra meals frozen. This makes subsequent meal prep quicker as some meals for the next week are already prepared. Consider prepping two weeks at a time, which is doable with big batch cooking.

Zero waste—The goal is to portion the food equally so nothing is left over. Because the preps use ingredients more than once, you shouldn't have leftover ingredients. It's always fine to add more vegetables than the recipe calls for. Vegetables add few macros, so more won't impact your fitness goals negatively.

What to freeze—Freeze any meal that you can't eat within five days. This ensures meals stay fresh and safe.

The best ways to reheat—The microwave is a time-saver, but reheating meals correctly takes a little finesse if you want them to taste good and have the right texture. Reheat chilled items for 50 to 60 seconds at a time, testing and rotating between each cooking increment. Let it rest a minute before eating. Reheat frozen items for the first two minutes at 50 percent power, then follow the directions for chilled items. If an item has any type of bread (breakfast sandwich, pancakes, etc.) wrap it in a damp paper towel before heating. This keeps it soft and prevents it from drying out.

TRACKING YOUR PROGRESS

As a nutritional and fitness coach, I stress to my clients the importance of establishing realistic and well-defined goals as well as collecting data in order to track their progress toward those goals. A powerful acronym that's been around for a while is SMART goal setting/tracking:

Specific—Establish exact perimeters such, as lose five pounds, eat eight servings of vegetables each day, or work out five times each week.

Measurable—Goals can be measured with data.

Achievable—Goals are realistic given the time period involved and with any limiting factors considered.

Relevant—The goal is relevant to your overall fitness aspirations.

Time bound—A good goal has a time frame, such as lose five pounds in one month or meal prep 20 days this month.

Your meal prep should facilitate those goals. If you aren't achieving your goals with meal prep, you need to make adjustments, such as increasing or decreasing your serving amounts a tad. Or switching to the strength training plan instead of the mixed cardio/strength plan. Keep track of your goals and data using a spreadsheet or one of the many great smartphone apps available.

About the Meal Prep Plans

This book has six weeks' worth of meal preps divided by the type of fitness you do: two weekly meal prep plans for cardio activities, two preps for strength activities, and two preps that focus on a combination of cardio and strength. It's important to note that you aren't locked into one particular regimen, and it's fine to use different preps as your fitness routine changes.

Each meal prep has everything you need to accomplish the prep successfully. It gives you the schedule, shopping list, equipment needed, strategies for cooking and prepping, and step-by-step cooking directions.

About the Recipes and Labels

The meal preps can be repeated as often as you want, but they're designed to get you started, provide a template for moving forward, and be a tool for developing your own meal preps, using your favorite recipes. No one wants to eat the same thing over and over again for weeks on end, so eventually you'll want to move beyond these meal preps and start getting a little creative. The preps are designed to feed one person for five days. Why five days and not seven? Five is the max amount of days food can be stored safely in the refrigerator, per USDA guidelines. The other two days can be supplemented with frozen prepped meals, once you get going. In part 3, I've included 42 more meal prep recipes that you can use to swap in or design your own weekly meal preps. All the recipes are labeled as strength, cardio, or cardio/strength so you'll know which ones can work where.

In addition to the fitness labels, each recipe will have additional labels (dairy-free, vegan, vegetarian, gluten-free, nut-free, pre-workout, and post-workout) that will be useful when choosing the recipe right for you, your dietary restrictions, and your fitness goals. Please check package labels carefully to ensure that gluten-free foods are produced in a gluten-free facility.

Each recipe also includes a reheat tip, because they're designed to be stored and eaten later. I'll share with you the best way to reheat each recipe from chilled or frozen.

Now it's time to get into the actual meal preps so you can put all this knowledge into practice. In the next three chapters, everything will be outlined in a step-by-step fashion. Feel free to skip to the chapter that aligns with your fitness routine and/or fitness goals.

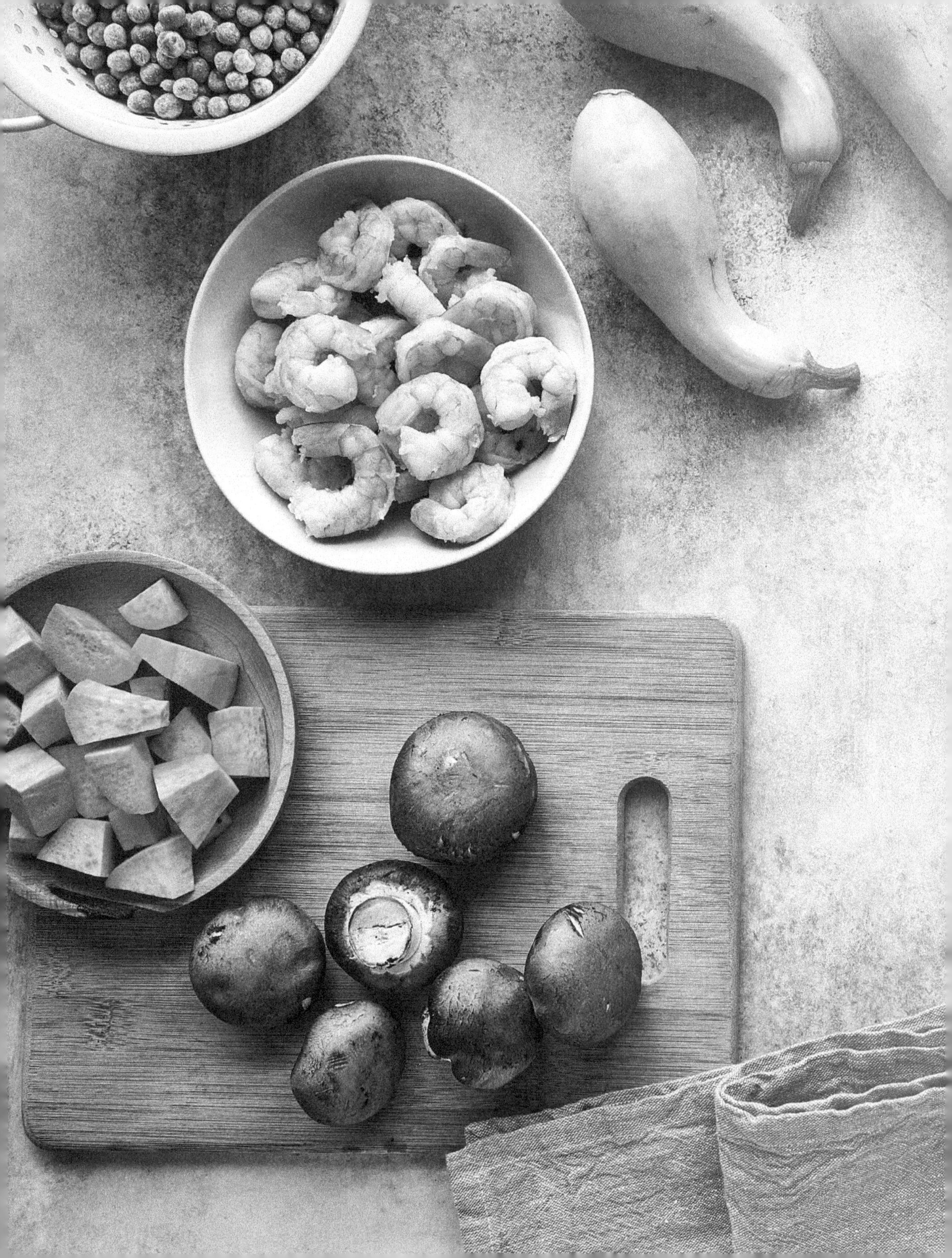

PART TWO

MEAL PREP FOR A FIT LIFESTYLE

In this part of the book, I'll outline six meal preps that you can use to fuel your cardio, strength training, or mixed workouts so you can be at the top of your game. The two preps in chapter 3 are for those who do mainly cardio activities, the two preps in chapter 4 are for people who mainly strength train, and the two preps in chapter 5 are for people who do a mix of both during the same workout or during a given week. Remember that these meal preps are designed to get you started. Feel free to mix and match to build your own meal preps. Many of the recipes can work for multiple exercise disciplines. Rest assured, you'll soon love the time meal prep saves you while still facilitating your fitness nutrition, and you'll love how it makes eating a whole foods–based diet so much easier.

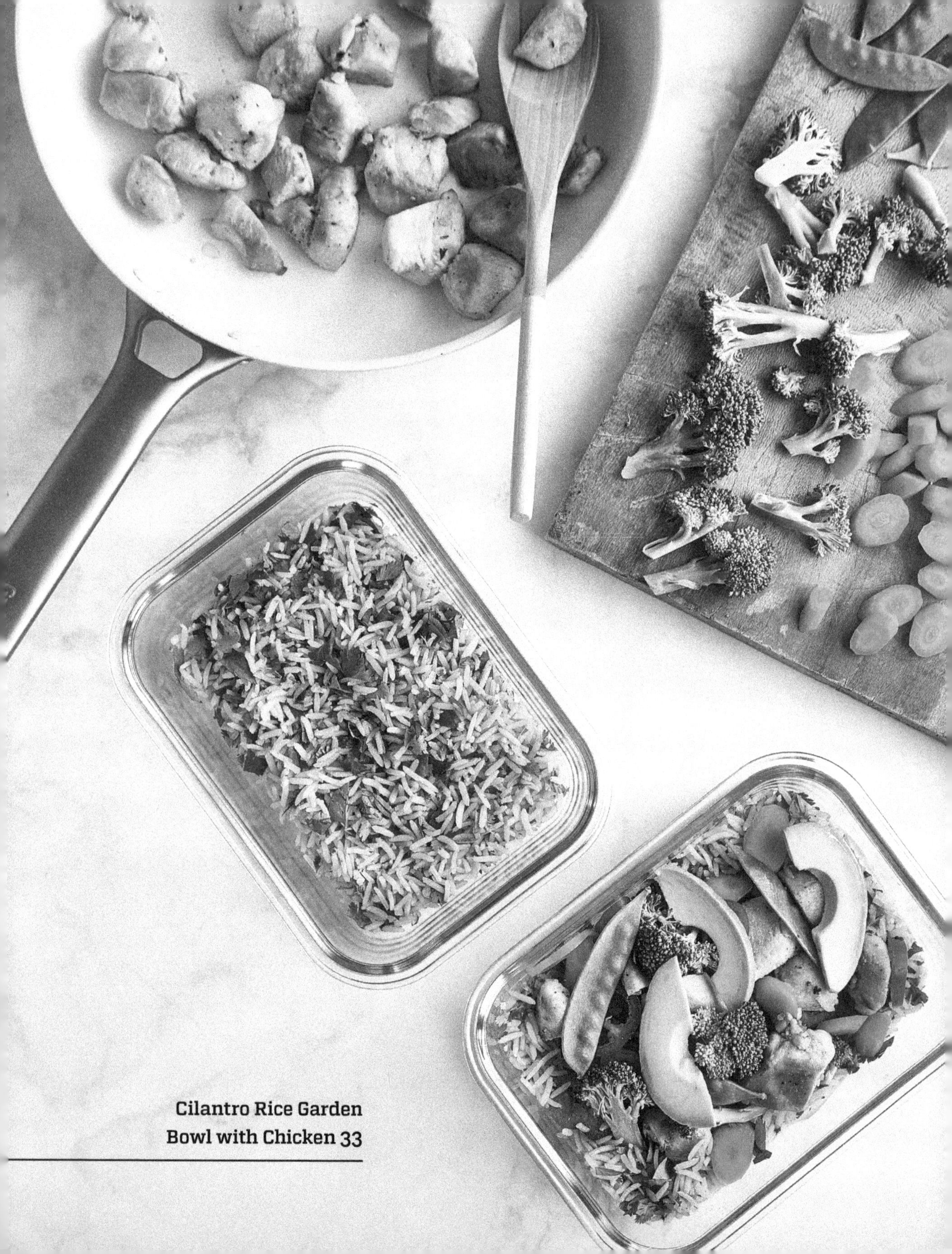

Cilantro Rice Garden Bowl with Chicken 33

CHAPTER THREE

MEAL PREPS FOR CARDIO

The following two meal preps are designed to fuel your cardio workouts. They focus on whole food–sourced complex carbs so your muscles will have the energy they need to go that extra mile and recover for the next workout. As a reminder, the serving sizes were developed with the nutritional needs of a 5'9", 175-pound man in mind, doing 45 to 60 minutes of cardio at least five times per week. You may have to adjust the serving sizes depending on your exact stats and needs. (See Calculating Your Daily Macros, page 5, for how to calculate your unique energy needs.)

PREP 1

Teriyaki Chicken Stir-Fry (page **32**)

Cilantro Rice Garden Bowl with Chicken (page **33**)

Savory Lentil Curry with Brown Rice (page **36**)

Hearty Sweet Potato Bowl with Panfried Tilapia (page **38**)

Overnight Blueberry Steel-Cut Oats (page **40**)

PREP 2

Walnut Chicken Stir-Fry with Brown Rice (page **44**)

Chicken Yum Bowl (page **46**)

Classic Red Beans and Rice (page **48**)

Hearty Veggie Power Bowl (page **50**)

Quinoa Porridge Breakfast Bowl (page **52**)

Mixed Berry Yogurt Parfait (page **53**)

Cardio Prep 1

This first prep is designed to help get your feet wet when it comes to meal prep. It consists of five easy-to-make meals. You'll start your day with some overnight oats and then lunches and dinners will be either a garden bowl with chicken, sweet potato bowl with tilapia, a chicken stir-fry, or a vegetarian curry. This week focuses on the power of brown rice as an excellent complex carb source that's easy to digest, economical, and a whole grain. Don't worry, I'm not forgetting about protein or fat; you'll get a balanced serving of those macros, too.

	BREAKFAST	LUNCH	WORKOUT/ REST	SNACK(S)	DINNER
MONDAY	Overnight Blueberry Steel-Cut Oats (page 40)	Teriyaki Chicken Stir-Fry (page 32)	Workout	1 banana, 1 apple, and 1 energy bar	Hearty Sweet Potato Bowl with Panfried Tilapia (page 38)
TUESDAY	Overnight Blueberry Steel-Cut Oats	Hearty Sweet Potato Bowl with Panfried Tilapia	Workout	1 banana, 1 apple, and 1 energy bar	Teriyaki Chicken Stir-Fry
WEDNESDAY	Overnight Blueberry Steel-Cut Oats	Cilantro Rice Garden Bowl with Chicken (page 33)	Rest	1 apple	Savory Lentil Curry with Brown Rice (page 36)
THURSDAY	Overnight Blueberry Steel-Cut Oats	Hearty Sweet Potato Bowl with Panfried Tilapia	Workout	1 banana, 1 apple, and 1 energy bar	Teriyaki Chicken Stir-Fry
FRIDAY	Overnight Blueberry Steel-Cut Oats	Cilantro Rice Garden Bowl with Chicken	Workout	1 banana, 1 apple, and 1 energy bar	Savory Lentil Curry with Brown Rice

Prep 1 Shopping List

Pantry

- Black pepper, freshly ground
- Cinnamon, ground
- Coconut oil
- Curry powder
- Garlic powder
- Honey (or agave, brown sugar, or coconut sugar)
- Lentils, dried green (1½ cups)
- Oats, quick-cook steel-cut (2½ cups)
- Olive oil cooking spray
- Sea salt
- Teriyaki sauce (1 cup)
- Vegetable stock (2 cups)

Produce

- Apples (5)
- Avocado (1 medium)
- Bananas (4)
- Broccoli florets (8 cups)
- Carrots, baby (1 [16-ounce] bag)
- Cilantro, fresh (1 bunch)
- Lime (1)
- Onions, yellow (2 medium)
- Snow peas (2 [8-ounce] bags)
- Spinach, baby (8 cups)
- Sweet mini peppers (16)
- Sweet potatoes (8 medium [4 to 5 inch] or 4 large [7 to 8 inch])

Protein

- Chicken, boneless, skinless breasts (3 pounds 6 ounces)
- Tilapia fillets (24 ounces)

Dairy

- 2% milk or milk alternative (2¼ cups)

Grains

- Rice, brown, uncooked (4½ cups)

Nuts and Seeds

- Walnuts, chopped (1 cup)

Other

- Blueberries, frozen (2 cups)

Equipment and Storage Vessels

- 2-quart pot with lid
- 5-quart pot with lid
- Chef's knife
- Cutting boards (2)
- Fork
- Glass meal prep containers with lids, large single-compartment (15)
- Large cast-iron skillet
- Large nonstick skillet
- Measuring cups and spoons
- Spatula
- Wooden spoons

Step-by-Step Prep

1. In a 5-quart pot, cook all the rice for the Teriyaki Chicken Stir-Fry, step 1 (page 32); Cilantro Rice Garden Bowl with Chicken, step 1 (page 33); and Savory Lentil Curry with Brown Rice, step 1 (page 36).
2. While the rice cooks, follow step 1 of the Hearty Sweet Potato Bowl with Panfried Tilapia (page 38) to cook the sweet potatoes.
3. While the rice and sweet potatoes cook, prep all the vegetables for the Teriyaki Chicken Stir-Fry, Cilantro Rice Garden Bowl with Chicken, Hearty Sweet Potato Bowl with Panfried Tilapia, and Savory Lentil Curry with Brown Rice.
4. Next, on a separate cutting board, cube all the chicken for the Cilantro Rice Garden Bowl with Chicken and Teriyaki Chicken Stir-Fry.
5. Use a cast-iron skillet to complete steps 3 through 5 of the Teriyaki Chicken Stir-Fry, using 2 pounds of the cubed chicken.
6. When that recipe is complete, cook the remaining chicken in a nonstick skillet following steps 3 through 8 of the Cilantro Rice Garden Bowl with Chicken.
7. Next, use the nonstick skillet to cook the tilapia and complete steps 4 through 7 of the Hearty Sweet Potato Bowl with Panfried Tilapia. While the tilapia is cooking, complete steps 2 and 3 of the recipe to mash the sweet potatoes.
8. The rice should be done and divided at this stage, so now use the 5-quart pot to follow steps 1 and 2 of the Savory Lentil Curry with Brown Rice.
9. While the lentil curry is cooking, completely prepare the Overnight Blueberry Steel-Cut Oats (page 40) recipe.
10. Complete steps 4 and 5 of the Savory Lentil Curry with Brown Rice.

Teriyaki Chicken Stir-Fry

CARDIO, DAIRY-FREE, GLUTEN-FREE, STRENGTH/CARDIO

PREP TIME: 15 MINUTES / **COOK TIME:** 40 MINUTES • **MAKES 3 SERVINGS**

This meal is complete with a boost of healthy carbs, protein, and a variety of fresh vegetables, plus the teriyaki sauce adds great flavor but not many calories. If you're looking for a teriyaki sauce, I recommend the Mr. Yoshida's brand. Remember that stir-fries are meant to cook fast and on higher heat to keep the vegetables on the crisp side.

2 cups brown rice, rinsed well
4 cups water
½ teaspoon sea salt
1 tablespoon coconut oil
2 pounds boneless, skinless chicken breast, cut into 1-inch cubes
1 medium onion, thinly sliced
16 baby carrots, sliced horizontally
4 cups coarsely chopped broccoli florets
1 (8-ounce) bag snow peas
8 sweet mini peppers, thinly sliced
¾ cup prepared teriyaki sauce

1. In a 2- to 5-quart pot over high heat, combine the rice, water, and salt and bring to a boil.
2. Turn the burner to low, stir a few times, cover, and let cook for about 40 minutes, until the water is absorbed.
3. While the rice is cooking, heat a large cast-iron skillet over medium-high heat. Pour in the oil, add the chicken, and cook, stirring, for about 5 minutes, until the chicken is cooked through and no longer pink.
4. Add the onion, carrots, broccoli, snow peas, and peppers. Cook, stirring every few seconds, for about 10 minutes, or until the vegetables are as soft as you prefer, then turn off the heat.
5. Evenly divide the rice into 3 single-compartment containers. Divide the chicken and vegetables evenly. Drizzle ¼ cup of teriyaki sauce over each and cover. Store in the fridge until needed.

Reheat: From the refrigerator, with the lid cracked, reheat in the microwave for 1 minute. Check, rotate, and cook for 1 more minute.

Per serving: Calories: 1,067, Total fat: 16g, Total carbs: 139g, Sugar: 25g, Protein: 89g, Fiber: 12g, Sodium: 4,283mg

Cilantro Rice Garden Bowl with Chicken

CARDIO, DAIRY-FREE, GLUTEN-FREE, NUT-FREE, STRENGTH/CARDIO, VEGAN OPTION

PREP TIME: 15 MINUTES / **COOK TIME:** 40 MINUTES • **MAKES 2 SERVINGS**

This bowl is packed with healthy carbs and micronutrients that will fuel your workouts and keep you feeling satisfied for hours. The suggested vegetables work great and are designed to use along with the other recipes for this week, but feel free to get creative and experiment with your own combinations.

1 cup brown rice, rinsed well
2 cups water
1 teaspoon sea salt, divided
22 ounces boneless, skinless chicken breast, cut into 1-inch cubes
2 teaspoons garlic powder
¼ teaspoon freshly ground black pepper
Olive oil cooking spray
½ cup chopped fresh cilantro
Juice of 1 lime
4 cups chopped broccoli florets
1 (8-ounce) bag fresh snow peas
8 sweet mini peppers, thinly sliced
16 baby carrots, thinly sliced
1 medium avocado, sliced

1. In a 2- to 5-quart pot over high heat, combine the rice, water, and ½ teaspoon of salt and bring to a boil.
2. Turn the burner to low, stir a few times, cover, and let cook for about 40 minutes, until water is absorbed.
3. While the rice is cooking, preheat a large nonstick skillet over medium heat.
4. Coat the chicken with the garlic powder, the remaining ½ teaspoon of salt, and the pepper.
5. Spray the skillet with cooking spray, then add the chicken. Gently sauté for 10 to 15 minutes, stirring every few minutes, until the chicken is cooked through and no longer pink. Set aside.

>>

Cilantro Rice Garden Bowl with Chicken continued

6. When the rice is cooked, add the cilantro and lime juice and stir until combined.
7. Evenly divide the rice into each of 4 single-compartment prep containers.
8. On top of the rice, divide the chicken, broccoli, snow peas, peppers, carrots, and avocado. Immediately cover the containers and place in the freezer. If you add the avocado later, you can store the containers in the refrigerator for up to 1 week.

Reheat: From frozen, with lid cracked, heat in the microwave for 2 minutes at 50 percent power and then an additional 2 minutes at full power. Allow to rest 1 minute before eating.

Substitution Tip: You can make this meal vegan by replacing the chicken with drained and rinsed canned chickpeas.

Per serving: Calories: 1,005, Total fat: 22g, Total carbs: 117g, Sugar: 16g, Protein: 88g, Fiber: 19g, Sodium: 1,438mg

Savory Lentil Curry with Brown Rice

CARDIO, GLUTEN-FREE, NUT-FREE, VEGAN

PREP TIME: 15 MINUTES / COOK TIME: 1 HOUR • MAKES 2 SERVINGS

This vegan recipe is packed with healthy carbs and a good dose of plant-based protein. The combination of lentils and rice delivers the essential amino acids to your body, which is great for muscle recovery. This curry is inspired by Indian flavors and is rich in turmeric, which has a lot of healthy properties, including reducing inflammation.

For the curry

1 tablespoon olive oil

1 medium onion, chopped into ½-inch pieces

3 tablespoons curry powder

1 tablespoon garlic powder

1 teaspoon sea salt

¼ teaspoon freshly ground black pepper

3 cups water

2 cups vegetable stock

1½ cups dried green lentils, rinsed

4 cups baby spinach

For the rice

1½ cups brown rice, rinsed well

3 cups water

¼ teaspoon sea salt

To make the curry

1. In a 5-quart pot over medium heat, heat the oil. Add the onion, curry powder, garlic powder, salt, and pepper and gently sauté for about 5 minutes, or until the onion is transluscent, stirring frequently.
2. Add the water, stock, lentils, and spinach. Increase the heat to high and bring to a full boil. Cover, reduce the heat to low, and simmer for about 50 minutes.

To make the rice

3. While the curry cooks, in a 2-quart pot over high heat, combine the rice, water, and salt. Bring to a full boil. Stir then turn the heat to low, cover, and cook for about 40 minutes, until water is absorbed.
4. Allow the lentils and rice to cool for 15 minutes once cooked.
5. Evenly divide the rice into each of 2 single-compartment prep containers. Top each container with half of the curry and cover. Store in the refrigerator until needed.

Reheat: From the refrigerator, with the lid cracked, heat in the microwave for 3 minutes, stirring after each 1-minute increment.

Per serving: Calories: 1,141, Total fat: 15g, Total carbs: 214g, Sugar: 9g, Protein: 45g, Fiber: 34g, Sodium: 2,113mg

Hearty Sweet Potato Bowl with Panfried Tilapia

CARDIO, GLUTEN-FREE, NUT-FREE, STRENGTH/CARDIO

PREP TIME: 15 MINUTES / **COOK TIME:** 30 MINUTES • **MAKES 3 SERVINGS**

Sweet potatoes are a perfect whole foods–based carb source that is flavorful and fiber rich. This recipe shows you an easy way to make sweet potatoes part of your regular diet to boost your nutrition and energy levels. If you aren't a fan of fish, you can easily make this recipe with chicken or another meat of your choice. If you like a sweet yet salty flavor, this recipe will be right up your alley.

4 cups water

4 large (or 8 medium) sweet potatoes, washed and cut into 1-inch cubes

¼ cup 2% milk or milk alternative

½ teaspoon sea salt

24 ounces frozen tilapia fillets

Olive oil cooking spray

1 tablespoon lemon pepper seasoning

3 cups baby spinach

1. Place the water in a 2- to 5-quart pot over high heat. Add the sweet potatoes and bring to a boil. Reduce the heat to medium and allow to cook, uncovered, for 25 to 30 minutes, or until the sweet potatoes are soft when stabbed with a fork.
2. Carefully drain the sweet potatoes using a lid or a colander.
3. Add the milk and salt and gently mash with a fork or a potato masher until uniform. (It's okay if it's a little lumpy.)
4. While the sweet potatoes are cooking, preheat a large nonstick skillet over medium heat.
5. Spray the fish fillets on both sides with cooking spray. Evenly sprinkle with the lemon pepper seasoning.
6. Spread the fillets out in the skillet and cover with a lid or baking tray. Cook for about 10 minutes, remove the lid, and turn each fillet. Cover and cook for about an additional 10 minutes. Turn the heat off and set aside.

7. Evenly divide the sweet potato into each of 3 single-compartment prep containers. Top each serving with 1 cup of spinach. Place equal amounts of tilapia on top of the spinach (about 8 ounces per container). Immediately seal each container with its lid and store in the refrigerator until needed.

Reheat: From the refrigerator, with the lid cracked, heat in the microwave for 2 to 3 minutes, stirring after each 1-minute increment. From frozen, with the lid cracked, heat in the microwave for 2 minutes at 50 percent power and then for an additional 2 to 3 minutes, stirring between minute increments.

Per serving: Calories: 665, Total fat: 7g, Total carbs: 78g, Sugar: 12g, Protein: 66g, Fiber: 11g, Sodium: 844mg

Overnight Blueberry Steel-Cut Oats

CARDIO, GLUTEN-FREE, VEGETARIAN

PREP TIME: 15 MINUTES • **MAKES 5 SERVINGS**

If you haven't tried steel-cut oats, you're in for a pleasant surprise. They aren't the sticky goo that you may think of when you hear the word oatmeal. Steel-cut oats have a completely different texture and make you feel fuller longer. This recipe lets your refrigerator do the work instead of your stove. You'll wake up to a bowl of morning deliciousness.

2 cups water
2 cups 2% milk or milk alternative
2½ cups quick-cook steel-cut oats
5 tablespoons honey (or agave, brown sugar, or coconut sugar)
Cinnamon
2 cups frozen blueberries
1 cup chopped walnuts

1. Evenly divide the water and milk into each of 5 single-compartment prep containers.
2. Add ½ cup of oats to each container and stir.
3. Stir 1 tablespoon of honey into each container.
4. Top each container with a pinch of cinnamon, one-fifth of the blueberries, and one-fifth of the walnuts and cover. Store in the refrigerator until needed.

Ingredient Tip: You can make this recipe using many different toppings so feel free to experiment with other fresh fruits, dried fruits, and nuts.

Reheat: This recipe can be eaten cold or warm. From the refrigerator, with the lid cracked, heat in the microwave for 1 minute.

Per serving: Calories: 594, Total fat: 23g, Total carbs: 97g, Sugar: 32g, Protein: 15g, Fiber: 12g, Sodium: 53mg

Cardio Prep 2

In this next cardio meal prep, we'll focus on another great whole foods–based carb source, the ancient grain quinoa. Quinoa is higher in protein than rice and offers more micronutrients. You'll start your day with a quinoa-based breakfast bowl and your lunches and dinners for the week will be a mix of beans and rice, chicken bowls, stir-fry, and a hearty vegetable bowl. Each day you'll also enjoy a parfait as a snack or a great pre- or post-workout option.

	BREAKFAST	LUNCH	WORKOUT/ REST	SNACK(S)	DINNER
MONDAY	Quinoa Porridge Breakfast Bowl (page 52)	Classic Red Beans and Rice (page 48)	Workout	Mixed Berry Yogurt Parfait (page 53) and 1 banana	Chicken Yum Bowl (page 46)
TUESDAY	Quinoa Porridge Breakfast Bowl	Walnut Chicken Stir-Fry with Brown Rice (page 44)	Workout	Mixed Berry Yogurt Parfait and 1 banana	Hearty Veggie Power Bowl (page 50)
WEDNESDAY	Quinoa Porridge Breakfast Bowl	Classic Red Beans and Rice	Rest	Mixed Berry Yogurt Parfait	Walnut Chicken Stir-Fry with Brown Rice
THURSDAY	Quinoa Porridge Breakfast Bowl	Walnut Chicken Stir-Fry with Brown Rice	Workout	Mixed Berry Yogurt Parfait and 1 banana	Hearty Veggie Power Bowl
FRIDAY	Quinoa Porridge Breakfast Bowl	Chicken Yum Bowl	Workout	Mixed Berry Yogurt Parfait and 1 banana	Classic Red Beans and Rice

Prep 2 Shopping List

Pantry

- Apple cider vinegar
- Beans, red (2 [15-ounce] cans)
- Beans, white (2 [15-ounce] cans)
- Cajun seasoning
- Cinnamon, ground
- Cornstarch
- Garlic powder
- Ginger, ground
- Honey (or agave or coconut sugar)
- Hot sauce
- Mayonnaise, light
- Oats, quick-cook steel-cut (1¼ cups)
- Oil, coconut
- Oil, olive
- Olive oil cooking spray
- Paprika
- Pepper, black
- Sea salt
- Soy sauce, reduced sodium
- Sugar, brown
- Tomato paste (1 can)
- Vanilla extract
- Vegetable stock (3 cups)

Produce

- Bananas (4)
- Bell peppers, green (2)
- Broccoli florets (4½ cups)
- Cauliflower (4½ cups)
- Celery (6 stalks)
- Cucumbers (2 medium)
- Lemon (1)
- Onions, yellow (2 medium)
- Spinach, baby (4 cups)
- Sweet mini peppers (15)
- Tomatoes, cherry (30)

Protein

- Chicken, boneless, skinless breasts (2½ pounds)

Dairy

- 2% milk or milk alternative (3 cups)
- Vanilla Greek yogurt or dairy-free yogurt (5 cups)

Grains

- Quinoa (2½ cups)
- Rice, brown (4 cups)

Nuts and Seeds

- Walnuts, chopped (1¼ cups)

Other

- Berries, mixed, frozen (5 cups)
- Cranberries, dried (1 cup)
- Tahini

Equipment and Storage Vessels

- 2-quart pot with lid
- 5-quart pot with lid
- Chef's knife
- Cutting boards (2)
- Fork
- Glass meal prep containers with lids, large single-compartment (20)
- Large cast-iron skillet
- Large nonstick skillet
- Measuring cups and spoons
- Mixing bowls
- Spatula
- Wooden spoons

Step-by-Step Prep

1. In a 5-quart pot, cook the rice for the Walnut Chicken Stir-Fry with Brown Rice (page 44), Chicken Yum Bowl (page 46), and Classic Red Beans and Rice (page 48).
2. While the rice is cooking, prep all the vegetables for the Walnut Chicken Stir-Fry with Brown Rice, Chicken Yum Bowl, Classic Red Beans and Rice, and Hearty Veggie Power Bowl (page 50).
3. Using a separate cutting board, cube the chicken for the Walnut Chicken Stir-Fry with Brown Rice and Chicken Yum Bowl.
4. Transfer the cooked rice to a bowl and use the 5-quart pot to complete steps 3 through 5 for the Classic Red Beans and Rice.
5. While the beans are cooking, use a 2-quart pot and follow steps 1 and 2 for the Hearty Veggie Power Bowl to cook the quinoa.
6. Complete steps 3 through 7 of the Walnut Chicken Stir-Fry with Brown Rice, then complete steps 3 through 8 of the Chicken Yum Bowl.
7. Complete steps 6 and 7 of the Classic Red Beans and Rice.
8. Rinse out the 5-quart pot and use it to complete steps 1 through 3 of the Quinoa Porridge Breakfast Bowl (page 52).
9. While the quinoa cooks, complete steps 3 through 5 of the Hearty Veggie Power Bowl.
10. Wrap things up by finishing steps 4 and 5 of the Quinoa Porridge Breakfast Bowl and complete all steps of for the Mixed Berry Yogurt Parfait (page 53).

Walnut Chicken Stir-Fry with Brown Rice

CARDIO, DAIRY-FREE, POST-WORKOUT, STRENGTH/CARDIO

PREP TIME: 15 MINUTES / COOK TIME: 40 MINUTES • MAKES 3 SERVINGS

This Chinese-inspired meal offers a trifecta of macronutrients. Lean protein from the chicken, complex carbs from the brown rice, and healthy fats from the walnuts provide what your body needs for fast recovery. This recipe is sure to be one you'll keep coming back to, not only because of its excellent nutrition but also because of its great flavor.

For the rice

1½ cups brown rice, rinsed well

3 cups water

½ teaspoon sea salt

For the sauce

½ cup water

5 teaspoons reduced-sodium soy sauce

3 tablespoons cornstarch

½ teaspoon ground ginger

2 teaspoons garlic powder

For the chicken and vegetables

1 tablespoon coconut oil

1½ pounds boneless, skinless chicken breast, cut into 1-inch cubes

1 medium onion, sliced

2 cups broccoli florets

2 cups cauliflower florets

2 celery stalks, thinly sliced

6 sweet mini peppers, thinly sliced

½ cup walnuts

To make the rice

1. In a 2- to 5-quart pot over high heat, combine the rice, water, and salt and bring to a boil.
2. Reduce the heat to low, stir a few times, cover, and cook for about 30 minutes, until the water is fully absorbed.

To make the sauce

3. In a small bowl, combine the water, soy sauce, cornstarch, ginger, and garlic powder. Stir and set aside.

To make the chicken and vegetables

4. Preheat a large cast-iron skillet over medium-high heat. Pour in the oil, add the chicken, and cook for about 5 minutes while stirring, until the chicken is no longer pink.
5. Add the onion, broccoli, cauliflower, celery, peppers, and walnuts and cook, stirring every few seconds, for 10 to 15 minutes, or until the vegetables are as soft as you prefer.
6. Stir the sauce and add it to the skillet. Keep stirring until the sauce thickens. Turn the heat off.
7. Evenly divide the rice into each of 3 single-compartment prep containers. Evenly divide the chicken and vegetables between the containers. Cover. Store in the refrigerator until needed.

Reheat: From the refrigerator, with the lid cracked, heat in the microwave for 3 minutes, stirring after each 1-minute increment.

Substitution Tip: Don't like walnuts? Use cashews or pecans instead.

Per serving: Calories: 548, Total fat: 24g, Total carbs: 28g, Sugar: 7g, Protein: 59g, Fiber: 6g, Sodium: 870mg

Chicken Yum Bowl

CARDIO, DAIRY-FREE, GLUTEN-FREE, NUT-FREE, POST-WORKOUT, STRENGTH/CARDIO

PREP TIME: 15 MINUTES / **COOK TIME:** 40 MINUTES • **MAKES 2 SERVINGS**

Bowls are a growing food trend because they combine several flavors and textures in one dish. They also focus on using fresh vegetables and whole-food ingredients. This recipe is no different. It will fuel your active day and give your body the micronutrients it needs for energy and optimum function.

For the rice

1 cup brown rice, rinsed well
2 cups water
Pinch sea salt

For the chicken and cooked vegetables

1 pound boneless, skinless chicken breast, cut into 1-inch cubes
1 tablespoon garlic powder
1 teaspoon sea salt
¼ teaspoon freshly ground black pepper
Olive oil cooking spray
1½ cups broccoli florets
1½ cups cauliflower florets

For the sauce

½ cup light mayonnaise
1 tablespoon apple cider vinegar
1 tablespoon tomato paste
1 teaspoon paprika
1 teaspoon garlic powder
1 tablespoon brown sugar
2 tablespoons water
1 teaspoon sea salt
¼ teaspoon freshly ground black pepper

For assembling

1 (15-ounce) can white beans, drained and rinsed
2 cups baby spinach
1 medium cucumber, thinly sliced
18 cherry tomatoes
9 sweet mini peppers, thinly sliced

To make the rice

1. In a 2-quart pot over high heat, combine the rice, water, and salt and bring to a full boil.

2. Reduce the heat to low, stir a few times, cover, and cook for about 30 minutes, until the water is fully absorbed.

To make the chicken and cooked vegetables

3. While the rice is cooking, preheat a large nonstick skillet over medium heat.
4. Coat the chicken with the garlic powder, salt, and pepper.
5. Spray the skillet with cooking spray and add the chicken. Gently sauté for 10 to 12 minutes, stirring every few minutes, until the chicken is cooked through and no longer pink.
6. While the chicken is cooking, cook the broccoli and cauliflower with a little water in a small microwave-safe bowl for 2 minutes in the microwave.

To make the sauce

7. In a small bowl, mix together the mayonnaise, vinegar, tomato paste, paprika, garlic powder, sugar, water, salt, and the pepper until smooth.

To assemble

8. Evenly divide the rice into 2 single-compartment containers. Top with the chicken, beans, and veggies, arranging each ingredient clockwise. Drizzle with sauce. Cover. Store in the refrigerator until needed.

Reheat: This bowl should be slightly warmed before eating. From the refrigerator, with the lid cracked, heat in the microwave for 1 minute.

Per serving: Calories: 1,190, Total fat: 26g, Total carbs: 161g, Sugar: 22g, Protein: 80g, Fiber: 30g, Sodium: 2,912mg

Classic Red Beans and Rice

CARDIO, GLUTEN-FREE, NUT-FREE, POST-WORKOUT, VEGAN

PREP TIME: 10 MINUTES / COOK TIME: 40 MINUTES • MAKES 3 SERVINGS

This Louisiana-inspired recipe is a healthier version of the typical red beans and rice you may have had before. Using canned beans makes this version speedy, and the combination of beans and rice gives your body the complete protein needed to recover from a good workout. This dish can be as spicy or mild as you like. Start with the given amount of hot sauce and add more to heat it up to your liking.

1½ cups brown rice, rinsed well
3 cups water
1 tablespoon olive oil
1 medium onion, cut into ½-inch dice
2 green bell peppers, cut into ¼-inch dice
4 celery stalks, thinly sliced
1 tablespoon garlic powder
1 tablespoon Cajun seasoning
2 tablespoons tomato paste
2 (15-ounce) cans red beans, drained and rinsed
3 cups vegetable stock
1½ teaspoons hot sauce
1 tablespoon sea salt

1. In a 2-quart pot over high heat, combine the rice and water and bring to a full boil.
2. Reduce the heat to low, stir a few times, cover, and cook for about 30 minutes, until water is fully absorbed.
3. In a 5-quart pot over medium heat, heat the oil. Add the onion, bell peppers, and celery and sauté for about 5 minutes, or until the vegetables are as soft as you prefer.
4. Add the garlic powder, Cajun seasoning, and tomato paste and stir until combined. Add the beans, stock, hot sauce, and salt.
5. Increase the heat to medium-high and, when the mixture comes to a slow boil, reduce the heat to medium-low and simmer for about 30 minutes.

6. Mash some of the beans with a spatula or fork to thicken.
7. Evenly divide the rice into 3 single-compartment prep containers. Pour one-third of the beans over the rice in each container. Cover. Store in the refrigerator until needed.

Reheat: From the refrigerator, with the lid cracked, heat in the microwave for 3 minutes, stirring after each 1-minute increment.

Per serving: Calories: 694, Total fat: 9g, Total carbs: 131g, Sugar: 9g, Protein: 25g, Fiber: 18g, Sodium: 3,551mg

Hearty Veggie Power Bowl

CARDIO, GLUTEN-FREE, NUT-FREE, PRE-WORKOUT, VEGAN

PREP TIME: 15 MINUTES / COOK TIME: 30 MINUTES • MAKES 2 SERVINGS

Many people think that vegan food is boring and bland, but that is far from the truth. Hopefully, this recipe will help convince you, if you still aren't sure. This bowl delivers a hefty dose of whole foods–based carbs and a nice serving of plant-based protein. Because the vegetables deliver a good dose of micronutrients, you'll be all set with this well-rounded vegan meal.

For the quinoa and cooked vegetables

1 cup quinoa, rinsed well
2 cups water
½ teaspoon sea salt
¼ teaspoon freshly ground black pepper
1 teaspoon garlic powder
1 cup broccoli florets
1 cup cauliflower florets

For the sauce

¼ cup prepared tahini
Juice of 1 lemon
1 teaspoon garlic powder
½ teaspoon sea salt
½ teaspoon paprika
3 tablespoons water

For assembling

1 (15-ounce) can white beans, drained and rinsed
2 cups baby spinach
12 cherry tomatoes
1 medium cucumber, thinly sliced

To make the quinoa and cooked vegetables

1. In a 2- to 5-quart pot over high heat, combine the quinoa, water, salt, pepper, and garlic powder. Bring to a boil, stirring every few seconds.
2. Once the mixture boils, turn the heat to low, stir once more, cover with a lid, and cook for about 20 minutes, or until the water is fully absorbed.
3. While the quinoa cooks, cook the broccoli and cauliflower with a little water in a small microwave-safe bowl for 2 minutes in the microwave.

To make the sauce

4. In a small bowl, combine the tahini, lemon juice, garlic powder, salt, and paprika. Stir. Add the water 1 tablespoon at a time until the sauce is pourable, adding more water if needed 1 tablespoon at a time.

To assemble

5. Evenly divide the quinoa into each of 2 single-compartment prep containers. In a clockwise fashion, evenly divide the broccoli/cauliflower, beans, spinach, tomatoes, and cucumber on top. Drizzle the sauce evenly over each bowl. Cover. Store in the refrigerator until needed.

Reheat: This bowl should be slightly warmed before eating. From the refrigerator, with the lid cracked, heat in the microwave for 1 minute.

Per serving: Calories: 822, Total fat: 24g, Total carbs: 125g, Sugar: 16g, Protein: 33g, Fiber: 33g, Sodium: 1,269mg

Quinoa Porridge Breakfast Bowl

CARDIO, GLUTEN-FREE, VEGETARIAN

PREP TIME: 5 MINUTES / **COOK TIME:** 30 MINUTES • **MAKES 5 SERVINGS**

You may think of quinoa as a side or for use in salads, but did you know it also makes a great breakfast porridge? Its nutty flavor complements a little sweetness, and there's no end to the fruit and nut mix-ins you can use. Quinoa is higher in protein than other breakfast grains and has a different, satisfying texture.

1½ cups quinoa, rinsed well
3 cups water
3 cups 2% milk or milk alternative
½ teaspoon sea salt
3 tablespoons honey (or agave, brown sugar, or coconut sugar)
1 teaspoon vanilla extract
2 teaspoons ground cinnamon
1 cup dried cranberries
¾ cup chopped walnuts

1. In a 5-quart pot over medium-high heat, combine the quinoa, water, milk, and salt. Bring to a boil, stirring every few seconds.
2. Turn the heat to low, stir once more, and cover with a lid. Cook for about 20 minutes, or until water is fully absorbed.
3. Stir in the honey, vanilla, cinnamon, and cranberries.
4. Immediately evenly divide the mixture into each of 5 single-compartment prep containers. (The mixture may be runny but will thicken as it sits.)
5. Sprinkle each container equally with the walnuts and cover. Store in the refrigerator until needed.

Reheat: This recipe can be eaten cold or warm. From the refrigerator, with the lid cracked, heat in the microwave for 1 minute.

Substitution Tip: Don't like walnuts? Use almonds, cashews, or hazelnuts instead.

Per serving: Calories: 532, Total fat: 18g, Total carbs: 83g, Sugar: 47g, Protein: 14g, Fiber: 8g, Sodium: 311mg

Mixed Berry Yogurt Parfait

CARDIO, GLUTEN-FREE, NUT-FREE, PRE-WORKOUT, STRENGTH/CARDIO, VEGETARIAN

PREP TIME: 10 MINUTES • **MAKES 5 SERVINGS**

In this recipe, the creaminess of the vanilla Greek yogurt pairs perfectly with the mixed berries, giving the dish a dessert-like feel, although it's actually a nutritious snack. This parfait offers a great way to fuel your workout without being too heavy or too sugary.

1¼ cups quick-cook steel-cut oats

5 cups frozen mixed berries

5 cups vanilla Greek yogurt or vanilla dairy-free yogurt alternative

1. Put ⅛ cup of oats into each of 5 single-compartment prep containers.
2. Top with ½ cup of berries in each container.
3. Then put ½ cup of yogurt on top of the berries.
4. Repeat steps 1 to 3 to use all the ingredients.
5. Cover. Store in the refrigerator until needed.

Substitution Tip: Feel free to experiment with other frozen or fresh fruits.

Per serving: Calories: 460, Total fat: 10g, Total carbs: 69g, Sugar: 31g, Protein: 26g, Fiber: 7g, Sodium: 100mg

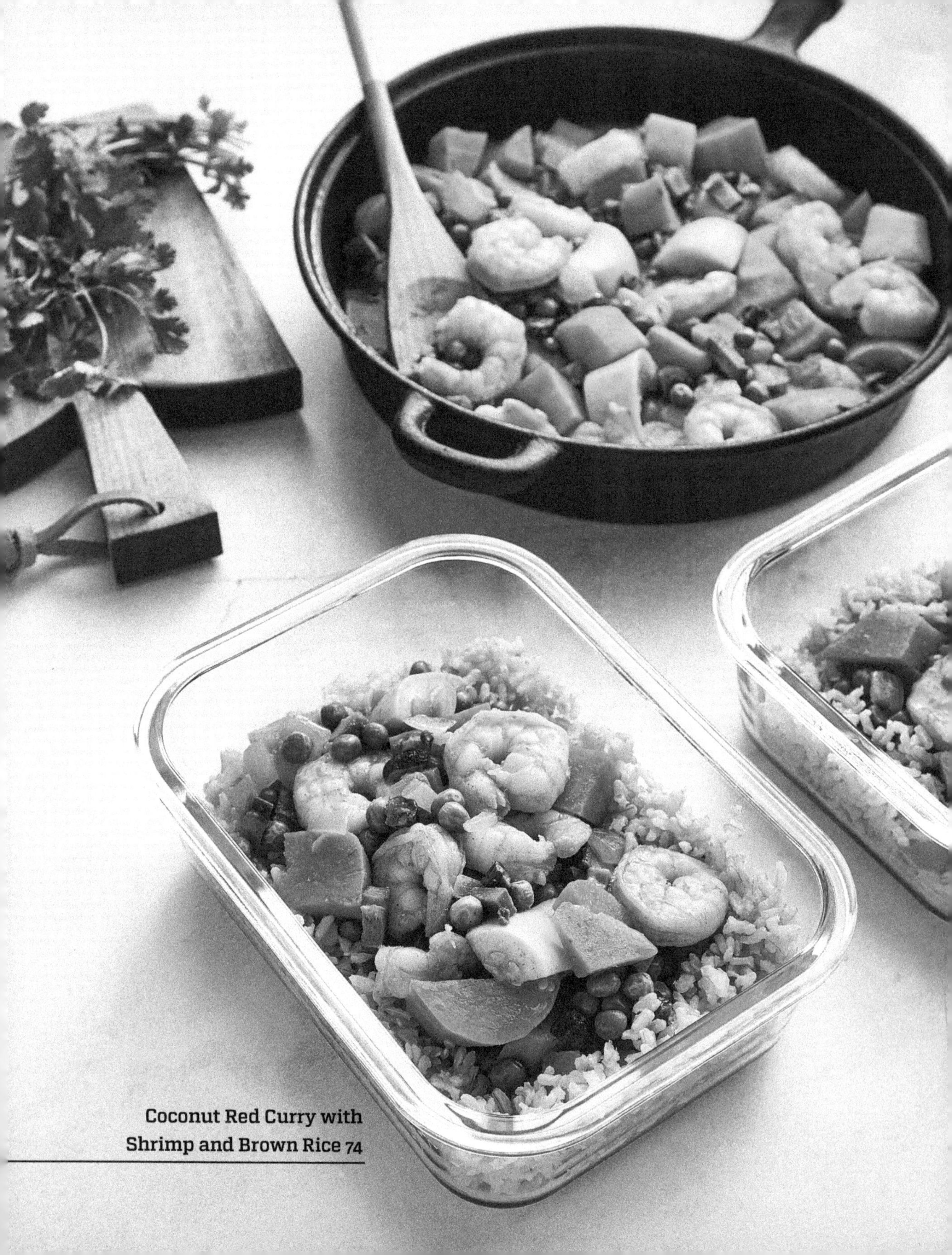

Coconut Red Curry with Shrimp and Brown Rice 74

CHAPTER FOUR

MEAL PREPS FOR STRENGTH

The two meal preps in this chapter are designed to fuel your strength training workouts with whole food–sourced protein and carbs. As a reminder, the serving sizes were developed for the nutritional needs of a 5'9" 175-pound man doing 45 to 60 minutes of strength training at least four times per week, so you may have to adjust the serving sizes, depending on your exact stats and needs. (See Calculating Your Daily Macros, page 5, for how to calculate your unique energy needs.)

PREP 1

PREP 2

Strength Prep 1

This strength-training meal prep teaches you how to make some easy protein-rich meals to ensure that your workouts will not be in vain. It consists of five protein-rich meals and some grab-and-go snacks, including a protein shake to consume after training. You'll start each morning with egg and sausage bites and then lunches and dinners will be either salmon burgers, chicken Parm, a stir-fry, or savory beef stew. This week focuses on a variety of protein sources, including some plant-based protein from chickpea pasta.

	BREAKFAST	LUNCH	WORKOUT/ REST	SNACK(S)	DINNER
MONDAY	Egg and Sausage Bites (page 65)	Salmon Burgers with Spring Greens (page 66)	Workout	1 banana, 1 apple, and 1 protein shake	Peanut Stir-Fried Noodles with Shrimp (page 62)
TUESDAY	Egg and Sausage Bites	One-Pot Savory Beef Stew (page 64)	Workout	1 banana, 1 apple, and 1 protein shake	Easy Chicken Parm with High-Protein Pasta (page 60)
WEDNESDAY	Egg and Sausage Bites	Salmon Burgers with Spring Greens	Rest	1 apple	Peanut Stir-Fried Noodles with Shrimp
THURSDAY	Egg and Sausage Bites	One-Pot Savory Beef Stew	Workout	1 banana, 1 apple, and 1 protein shake	Easy Chicken Parm with High-Protein Pasta
FRIDAY	Egg and Sausage Bites	Peanut Stir-Fried Noodles with Shrimp	Workout	1 banana, 1 apple, and 1 protein shake	One-Pot Savory Beef Stew

Prep 1 Shopping List

Pantry

- Apple cider vinegar
- Beef gravy packets (2)
- Bread crumbs, Italian-style (15 ounces)
- Garlic powder
- Honey (or agave, brown sugar, or coconut sugar)
- Hot sauce (optional)
- Oil, coconut
- Oil, olive
- Olive oil cooking spray
- Marinara sauce (24 ounces)
- Mayonnaise, light
- Mustard, Dijon
- Paprika
- Peanut butter, natural
- Pepper, black
- Sea salt
- Soy sauce, reduced-sodium

Produce

- Apples (5)
- Bananas (4)
- Carrots, baby (1 [32-ounce] bag)
- Lemon (1)
- Lime (1)
- Onions, yellow (2 medium)
- Potatoes, yellow (3 pounds)
- Spinach, baby (3 cups)
- Spring salad mix, organic (16 cups)
- Sweet mini peppers (11)
- Tomatoes, cherry (12)

Protein

- Beef, lean sirloin (1 pound)
- Chicken, boneless, skinless breasts (10 ounces)
- Salmon (1 [14.75-ounce] can)
- Shrimp, frozen, peeled, deveined, tail-off precooked (1½ pounds)
- Turkey sausage patties, precooked (5)

Dairy

- 2% milk or milk alternative (½ cup)
- Cheese, shredded Parmesan (½ cup)
- Cheese, shredded sharp cheddar (1 cup)
- Eggs (5 large)
- Egg whites, in carton (2½ cups)

Grains

- Bread, whole-grain (7 slices)
- Pasta, chickpea, vermicelli or linguine (18 ounces)

Nuts and Seeds

- Peanuts, chopped (¼ cup)

Other

- Mixed stir-fry vegetables, frozen (6 cups)
- Peas, frozen (2 cups)
- Protein shakes (4 [~30 grams protein])

Equipment and Storage Vessels

- 5-quart pot with lid
- Baking sheet
- Blender
- Chef's knife
- Colander
- Cutting boards (2)
- Glass meal prep containers with lids, large double-compartment (2)
- Glass meal prep containers with lids, large single-compartment (15)
- Large cast-iron skillet
- Large nonstick skillet
- Mason jars or small containers (2)
- Measuring cups and spoons
- Mixing bowls
- Muffin pan
- Parchment paper
- Spatula
- Whisk
- Wooden spoons

Step-by-Step Prep

1. Because three recipes call for a 5-quart pot, start your prep by cooking the chickpea pasta for both Easy Chicken Parm with High-Protein Pasta (step 5, page 60) and Peanut Stir-Fried Noodles with Shrimp (step 2, page 62). Once cooked, drain in a colander and rinse with hot water. Set aside.
2. Using the 5-quart pot, complete steps 1 through 3 of One-Pot Savory Beef Stew (page 64).
3. Preheat the oven to 375°F. Complete steps 1 through 4 of Easy Chicken Parm with High-Protein Pasta and steps 1 through 5 of Egg and Sausage Bites (page 65). Put both in the oven at the same time, but remove the Egg and Sausage Bites after 25 minutes, then finish the bites (steps 6 and 7).

4. Next, complete steps 4 and 5 of One-Pot Savory Beef Stew after the first 45 minutes are done.
5. While the One-Pot Savory Beef Stew is simmering, complete step 1 and steps 3 through 6 of Peanut Stir-Fried Noodles with Shrimp and steps 6 and 7 of Easy Chicken Parm with High-Protein Pasta.
6. Prepare the Salmon Burgers with Spring Greens (page 66) fully.
7. At this stage, the One-Pot Savory Beef Stew should be about finished. (If the timer has gone off prior, simply turn the heat off and allow it to sit until you're ready.) Complete the remaining steps 6 to 8.

Easy Chicken Parm with High-Protein Pasta

NUT-FREE, POST-WORKOUT, STRENGTH

PREP TIME: 15 MINUTES / **COOK TIME:** 40 MINUTES • **MAKES 2 SERVINGS**

I love Italian-inspired food; the flavors, textures, and aromas are so comforting. However, many dishes in this category can be high in fat, carbs, and saturated fat. Therefore, one of my favorite things to do in the kitchen is make healthier versions of Italian classics. This recipe has all the deliciousness of classic chicken Parmesan and pasta but with less fat, carbs, and saturated fat. It delivers a hefty dose of protein to help you recover from your workouts faster.

Olive oil cooking spray
1 cup Italian-style bread crumbs
½ cup finely shredded Parmesan cheese, divided
½ teaspoon garlic powder
¼ teaspoon sea salt
¼ teaspoon freshly ground black pepper
1 large egg
2 (5-ounce) boneless, skinless chicken breasts, butterflied into 4 thin fillets
8 cups water
8 ounces chickpea pasta
1 (24-ounce) jar marinara sauce

1. Preheat the oven to 375°F. Line a baking sheet with parchment paper and spray lightly with cooking spray.
2. In a shallow bowl, combine the bread crumbs, ¼ cup of Parmesan, the garlic powder, salt, and pepper. In another shallow bowl, beat the egg.
3. Dip each chicken fillet first in the egg, then coat both sides with the bread crumb mixture. Place on the prepared baking sheet.
4. Place the sheet in the oven and cook for about 35 minutes, or until a thermometer reads 165°F.
5. In a 5-quart pot, bring the water to a boil. When there's about 10 minutes of cooking time left for the chicken, add the pasta to the boiling water, stir, and cook for about 10 minutes, or until al dente. Drain in a colander and rinse with hot tap water.

6. When the oven timer goes off, remove the baking sheet from the oven, place 1 tablespoon of marinara on each fillet, and top each with equal amounts of the remaining ¼ cup of Parmesan. Return to the oven for about 5 minutes, or until the cheese is melted.
7. Place half the pasta and 2 chicken fillets in each of 2 divided meal prep containers. Top the pasta with equal amounts of the remaining marinara. Let cool for 5 minutes. Cover. Store in the refrigerator or freezer until needed.

Ingredient Tip: I've found the Banza brand of chickpea pasta has the taste and texture of traditional dry pasta.

Reheat: From the refrigerator, with the lid cracked, heat in the microwave for about 2 minutes, stirring after each 1-minute increment.

Per serving: Calories: 1,121, Total fat: 29g, Total carbs: 143g, Sugar: 34g, Protein: 81g, Fiber: 20g, Sodium: 2,973mg

Peanut Stir-Fried Noodles with Shrimp

DAIRY-FREE, STRENGTH, STRENGTH/CARDIO

PREP TIME: 10 MINUTES / COOK TIME: 15 MINUTES • MAKES 3 SERVINGS

This high-protein Southeast Asian–inspired meal is a great way to recover from a good lifting session. The peanut butter adds a lot of flavor and the noodles make the meal filling. Shrimp is an often-overlooked protein source, but it's a great lean option.

For the sauce

½ cup natural peanut butter
2 tablespoons reduced-sodium soy sauce
2 tablespoons honey (or agave or brown sugar)
¼ teaspoon hot sauce (optional)
Juice of 1 lime
¼ cup water

For the stir-fry

10 ounces uncooked chickpea pasta (linguini or vermicelli)
1 tablespoon coconut oil
6 cups frozen mixed stir-fry vegetables
1 tablespoon garlic powder
1½ pounds frozen, peeled, deveined, tail-off precooked shrimp
¼ cup chopped peanuts

To make the sauce

1. In a small bowl, combine the peanut butter, soy sauce, honey, hot sauce (if using), lime juice, and water and stir together until smooth. Set aside.

To make the stir-fry

2. Bring a 5-quart pot filled halfway with water to a boil over high heat. Add the pasta and cook for about 8 minutes, or until al dente. Drain the pasta in a colander.

3. While the pasta is cooking, pour the oil into a large cast-iron skillet over medium-high heat. Immediately add the frozen vegetables and stir until thawed and hot, about 5 minutes.

4. Add the garlic powder, shrimp, and peanuts. Continue cooking until the shrimp have thawed and are hot, about 10 minutes.

5. Turn off the burner and add the cooked pasta and peanut sauce. Mix until well combined.

6. Evenly divide the mixture into each of 3 single-compartment prep containers. Cover. Store in the refrigerator until needed.

Reheat: From the refrigerator, with the lid cracked, heat in the microwave for 3 minutes, stirring gently after each 1-minute increment.

Per serving: Calories: 1,015, Total fat: 39g, Total carbs: 96g, Sugar: 28g, Protein: 85g, Fiber: 16g, Sodium: 1,185mg

One-Pot Savory Beef Stew

DAIRY-FREE, NUT-FREE, POST-WORKOUT, PRE-WORKOUT, STRENGTH

PREP TIME: 15 MINUTES / **COOK TIME:** 1 HOUR 35 MINUTES • **MAKES 3 SERVINGS**

Nothing says comfort food like a big bowl of beef stew. The key to making beef stew healthier is choosing a lean cut. The goal is to cook the beef long enough for the collagen to break down, which results in very tender meat.

1 pound lean beef, cut into 1-inch cubes
8 cups water, divided
1 medium onion, chopped
2 tablespoons garlic powder
¼ teaspoon freshly ground black pepper
1 (16-ounce) bag baby carrots
3 pounds yellow potatoes, unpeeled, cut into 1- to 2-inch cubes
2 cups frozen peas
2 beef gravy packets

1. In a 5-quart pot over medium-high heat, sear the beef until the outside edges are light brown, about 5 minutes.
2. Add 7 cups of water, the onion, garlic powder, and pepper, and bring the mixture to a boil.
3. Reduce the heat to low, cover, and let simmer for about 45 minutes.
4. Add the carrots, potatoes, and peas. Increase the heat to medium-high and bring to a boil.
5. Reduce the heat to low, cover, and let simmer for about another 45 minutes, until the vegetables and beef are tender.
6. At the end of the cooking time, in a small bowl, whisk together the remaining 1 cup of water with the gravy packets until well dissolved. Stir into the stew.
7. Increase the heat to medium and bring to a boil, stirring to thicken. Turn off the heat and let cool for 15 minutes.
8. Evenly divide the stew into each of 3 single-compartment prep containers. Cover. Store in the refrigerator until needed.

Reheat: From the refrigerator, with the lid cracked, heat in the microwave for 3 minutes, stirring between each 1-minute increment.

Per serving: Calories: 835, Total fat: 10g, Total carbs: 146g, Sugar: 19g, Protein: 50g, Fiber: 14g, Sodium: 1,141mg

Egg and Sausage Bites

NUT-FREE, STRENGTH

PREP TIME: 10 MINUTES / **COOK TIME:** 25 MINUTES • **MAKES 10 BITES**

If you love eggs, sausage, and toast but just don't have time in the mornings to cook, this recipe will be right up your alley. It combines all the goodness of those items in a convenient portable package. This recipe gives your day a protein boost and a good balance of protein, carbs, and fat to help you feel satisfied throughout busy mornings.

5 large eggs

2½ cups carton egg whites

½ cup milk or milk alternative

7 slices whole-grain bread, cubed

5 precooked turkey sausage patties, crumbled

1 medium onion, cut into ¼-inch dice

3 cups coarsely chopped baby spinach

5 sweet mini peppers, cut into ¼-inch dice

½ teaspoon sea salt

¼ teaspoon freshly ground black pepper

1 cup shredded sharp cheddar cheese

Olive oil cooking spray

1. Preheat the oven to 375°F. In a medium bowl, whisk together the eggs, egg whites, and milk.
2. Stir in the bread, sausage, onion, spinach, sweet peppers, salt, black pepper, and cheese until the mixture is uniform and the bread looks wet.
3. Spray 10 wells of a nonstick muffin pan with cooking spray.
4. Divide the egg mixture evenly between the 10 wells.
5. Place in the oven on the middle rack and bake for about 25 minutes, or until the centers of the egg bites are set.
6. Remove from the oven and let cool for 10 to 15 minutes.
7. Place 2 egg bites in each of 5 meal prep containers. Cover. Store in the refrigerator until needed.

Reheat: From refrigerated, with the lid cracked, heat in the microwave for 45 seconds. Allow to rest another 45 seconds before eating.

Per serving (2 bites): Calories: 477, Total fat: 19g, Total carbs: 38g, Sugar: 11g, Protein: 38g, Fiber: 8g, Sodium: 1,124mg

Salmon Burgers with Spring Greens

NUT-FREE, POST-WORKOUT, STRENGTH

PREP TIME: 10 MINUTES / COOK TIME: 16 MINUTES • MAKES 2 SERVINGS

This low-carb meal gives you a great protein option to include on fresh salads. I always have a big tub of organic spring mix in the refrigerator, as it's a fast and easy way to get some green leafy vegetables in and to make a quick fresh salad. I include a homemade dressing that goes well with salmon, but feel free to use your favorite dressing. Salmon not only is a great protein choice but also contains healthy fats.

For the salmon

1 (14.75-ounce) can salmon
1 large egg
1 tablespoon light mayonnaise
Juice of ½ lemon
¼ cup Italian-style bread crumbs
½ teaspoon paprika
¼ teaspoon freshly ground black pepper
Olive oil cooking spray

For the dressing and salad

Juice of ½ lemon
¼ cup apple cider vinegar
2 tablespoons olive oil
1 tablespoon Dijon mustard
4 tablespoons honey
½ teaspoon sea salt
16 cups organic spring mix
12 cherry tomatoes
6 sweet mini peppers, thinly sliced
6 baby carrots, thinly sliced

To make the salmon

1. Heat a large nonstick skillet over medium heat.
2. Empty the salmon into a small bowl and remove the backbone only. Add the egg, mayonnaise, lemon juice, bread crumbs, paprika, and pepper. Stir together until well combined. Use a spoon to make 4 equal patties.

3. Spray the skillet with cooking spray. Add the salmon patties and cook for about 8 minutes, or until golden brown and crispy. Flip with a spatula and cook for about 8 more minutes.

To make the dressing and salad

4. In a blender, combine the lemon juice, vinegar, olive oil, mustard, honey, and salt and pulse until smooth.
5. Evenly divide the greens into each of 2 large prep containers. Top each container with even amounts of the tomatoes, peppers, and carrots. Cover and place in the refrigerator.
6. Divide the dressing between 2 small prep containers or small mason jars. Seal and place in the refrigerator. (Be sure to shake or stir before using). Place 2 salmon burgers into each of 2 separate containers. Cover and place in the refrigerator.

Prep Tip: This salad is designed to store well in the refrigerator for up to 1 week, but if you have time, you can make the salad fresh, right before you're ready to eat.

Reheat: Only the salmon will need to be heated, if you want it warm. From the refrigerator, with the lid cracked, heat in the microwave for 1 minute.

Per serving: Calories: 752, Total fat: 29g, Total carbs: 75g, Sugar: 44g, Protein: 59g, Fiber: 13g, Sodium: 2,063mg

Strength Prep 2

In this second strength meal prep we still focus on higher protein but also include a high-protein tuna snack for after your workout. You'll start each day with a filling burrito bowl and your lunches and dinners will alternate between four high-protein meals that are sure to help you build muscle and keep you feeling satisfied.

	BREAKFAST	LUNCH	WORKOUT/ REST	SNACK(S)	DINNER
MONDAY	Breakfast Burrito Bowl (page 76)	Oven Chicken, Spinach, and Mushroom Risotto (page 72)	Workout	Albacore Tuna Salad (page 81), 1 banana, and 1 apple	Black Bean Turkey Chili (page 78)
TUESDAY	Breakfast Burrito Bowl	Lemon Chicken with Quinoa and Spring Greens (page 79)	Workout	Albacore Tuna Salad, 1 banana, and 1 apple	Coconut Red Curry with Shrimp and Brown Rice (page 74)
WEDNESDAY	Breakfast Burrito Bowl	Black Bean Turkey Chili	Rest	Albacore Tuna Salad, 1 banana, 1 apple	Oven Chicken, Spinach, and Mushroom Risotto
THURSDAY	Breakfast Burrito Bowl	Lemon Chicken with Quinoa and Spring Greens	Workout	Albacore Tuna Salad, 1 banana, and 1 apple	Coconut Red Curry with Shrimp and Brown Rice
FRIDAY	Breakfast Burrito Bowl	Oven Chicken, Spinach, and Mushroom Risotto	Workout	Albacore Tuna Salad, 1 banana, and 1 apple	Black Bean Turkey Chili

Prep 2 Shopping List

Pantry

- Beans, black (2 [15-ounce] cans)
- Chicken broth (5 cups) or 5 bouillon cubes + water
- Chili seasoning (2 packets)
- Coconut milk, light (1 [13.5-ounce] can)
- Fish sauce
- Flour, whole wheat (or gluten-free)
- Garlic powder
- Hot sauce (optional)
- Mayonnaise, light
- Oil, olive
- Olive oil cooking spray
- Paprika
- Pepper, black
- Red curry paste
- Sea salt
- Taco seasoning
- Thyme, dried
- Tomatoes, diced (1 [28-ounce] can)
- Tortilla chips, baked (1 bag)

Produce

- Apples (4)
- Bananas (4)
- Carrots, baby (1 [16-ounce] bag)
- Cilantro, fresh (1 bunch)
- Lemons (2)
- Mushrooms, white button (3 cups)
- Onions, yellow (4 medium)
- Spinach, baby (13 cups)
- Spring salad mix, organic (16 cups)
- Squash, yellow (3 medium)
- Sweet mini peppers (11)
- Sweet potatoes (2 medium)
- Tomatoes, cherry (12)

Protein

- Chicken, boneless, skinless breasts (2½ pounds)
- Shrimp, frozen, peeled, deveined, tail-off precooked (1 pound)
- Tuna, solid white albacore (2 [12-ounce] cans)
- Turkey, ground, 92% lean (1 pound)
- Turkey, precooked sausage patties (5)

Dairy

- Cheese, 2% shredded Mexican style (1¼ cups)
- Cheese, shredded Parmesan (¾ cup)
- Egg whites, carton (1½ cups)
- Eggs (5 large)

Grains

- Crackers, whole-grain (20)
- Quinoa (1 cup)
- Rice, brown (3½ cups)

Other

- Peas, frozen (2 cups)

Equipment and Storage Vessels

- 2-quart pot with lid
- 5-quart pot with lid
- 9-by-13-inch baking dish
- Chef's knife
- Colander
- Cutting boards (2)
- Glass meal prep containers with lids, large single-compartment (15)
- Glass meal prep containers with lids, medium single-compartment (5)
- Glass meal prep containers with lids, small single-compartment (5) or resealable sandwich bags
- Large cast-iron skillet
- Large nonstick skillet
- Measuring cups and spoons
- Mixing bowls
- Parchment paper
- Spatula
- Wooden spoons

Step-by-Step Prep

1. Prepare steps 1 through 3 of the Oven Chicken, Spinach, and Mushroom Risotto (page 72).
2. While that's baking, use a 2-quart pot to complete steps 1 and 2 of the Coconut Red Curry with Shrimp and Brown Rice (page 74) to cook the rice.
3. Once the rice is simmering, prep all the vegetables for the Breakfast Burrito Bowl (page 76); Black Bean Turkey Chili (page 78); Lemon Chicken with Quinoa and Spring Greens (page 79); Coconut Red Curry with Shrimp and Brown Rice; and Oven Chicken, Spinach, and Mushroom Risotto.
4. Using a separate cutting board, cube the chicken breast for the Oven Chicken, Spinach, and Mushroom Risotto.
5. Use the 5-quart pot to complete steps 1 through 4 of the Black Bean Turkey Chili.

6. While the chili is cooking, use a nonstick skillet and 2-quart pot to completely prepare the Lemon Chicken with Quinoa and Spring Greens.
7. Use the cast-iron skillet to complete steps 3 through 5 of the Coconut Red Curry with Shrimp and Brown Rice.
8. When your nonstick skillet is free, complete the Breakfast Burrito Bowl.
9. At this stage, the Black Bean Turkey Chili and Oven Chicken Spinach, Mushroom, and Risotto should be cooked. Finish those recipes as directed.
10. Wrap things up by completely preparing Albacore Tuna Salad with Whole-Grain Crackers (page 81).

Oven Chicken, Spinach, and Mushroom Risotto

GLUTEN-FREE, NUT-FREE, POST-WORKOUT, STRENGTH, STRENGTH/CARDIO

PREP TIME: 15 MINUTES / **COOK TIME:** 45 MINUTES • **MAKES 3 SERVINGS**

Risotto is a one-pan rice dish that originated in Italy. It's basically a combination of protein, vegetables, seasonings, and rice. Because the rice is cooked in broth and seasonings, the rice absorbs all those flavors, making for a very flavorful dish. This recipe has been tweaked to be higher in protein than traditional risotto, while still having a nice dose of healthy carbs to recharge you after your workouts. It's also cooked in the oven so you can focus on other things while it's cooking.

4 cups chicken broth
2 cups brown rice, rinsed well
2 tablespoons olive oil
2 teaspoons garlic powder
1 teaspoon paprika
1 teaspoon sea salt
1½ pounds boneless, skinless chicken breasts, cut into 1-inch cubes
2 cups thinly sliced mushrooms
1 medium onion, cut into ¼-inch dice
6 cups coarsely chopped baby spinach
¼ teaspoon freshly ground black pepper
¾ cup grated Parmesan cheese

1. Preheat the oven to 375°F. Line a 9-by-13-inch baking dish with parchment paper.
2. In a large bowl, combine the broth, rice, oil, garlic powder, paprika, salt, chicken, mushrooms, onion, spinach, and pepper.
3. Pour the mixture into the prepared baking dish and place on the middle rack of the oven. Bake for about 45 minutes, or until the liquid is absorbed.
4. Remove from the oven and let cool for 15 minutes.

5. Evenly divide the risotto into each of 3 single-compartment prep containers. Top each with ¼ cup of Parmesan. Cover. Store in the refrigerator until needed.

Reheat: From the refrigerator, with the lid cracked, heat in the microwave for 3 minutes, stirring after each 1-minute increment.

Substitution Tip: If you don't like mushrooms, swap them out for any vegetable of your choice: frozen peas, broccoli florets, carrots, etc.

Per serving: Calories: 998, Total fat: 27g, Total carbs: 115g, Sugar: 5g, Protein: 74g, Fiber: 7g, Sodium: 2,625mg

Coconut Red Curry with Shrimp and Brown Rice

DAIRY-FREE, GLUTEN-FREE, STRENGTH, STRENGTH/CARDIO, VEGAN OPTION

PREP TIME: 15 MINUTES / **COOK TIME:** 40 MINUTES • **MAKES 2 SERVINGS**

This curry is so flavorful and a great way to enjoy lean protein and healthy carbs. Many people are intimidated when it comes to making curries because of all the herbs and spices needed. Luckily, red curry paste is now readily available in most grocery stores and contains all the herbs and spices you need. This meal offers a great way to refuel and recover from intense workouts.

1½ cups brown rice, rinsed well
3 cups water
1 can light coconut milk
1 tablespoon red curry paste (more if you like it spicy)
1 medium yellow squash, cut into 1-inch pieces
2 red sweet potatoes, cut into 1- to 2-inch pieces
1 medium onion, cut into ¼-inch dice
2 cups frozen peas
1 cup diced mushrooms
1 pound frozen peeled, deveined, tail-off precooked shrimp
1 tablespoon fish sauce
½ cup coarsely chopped fresh cilantro, for garnish (optional)

1. In a 2- to 5-quart pot over high heat, combine the rice and water. Bring to a boil.
2. Turn the heat to low, stir a few times, cover, and cook for about 40 minutes.
3. Preheat a large cast-iron skillet over medium-high heat. Pour in the coconut milk, curry paste, squash, sweet potatoes, onion, and peas. Bring to a slow boil and cook for about 10 minutes.
4. Reduce the heat to medium and add the mushrooms and shrimp. Cook for about 5 more minutes, or until the shrimp is thawed and heated through. Turn off the heat and stir in the fish sauce.

5. Evenly divide the rice into 2 single-compartment prep containers. Divide the curry evenly on top of the rice. Divide the cilantro (if using) on top of each. Cover. Store in the refrigerator until needed.

Reheat: From the refrigerator, with the lid cracked, heat in the microwave for 3 minutes, stirring after each 1-minute increment.

Substitution Tip: This meal can easily be made vegan by replacing the shrimp with a can of fava beans and omitting the fish sauce.

Per serving: Calories: 1,110, Total fat: 18g, Total carbs: 175g, Sugar: 19g, Protein: 60g, Fiber: 17g, Sodium: 2,021mg

Breakfast Burrito Bowl

GLUTEN-FREE, NUT-FREE, STRENGTH

PREP TIME: 10 MINUTES / **COOK TIME:** 20 MINUTES • **MAKES 5 SERVINGS**

For anyone who's ever spent time in the Southwest, breakfast burritos are a staple, and any local taco shop can have lines of people waiting to get their hands on this delicious morning meal. However, the typical breakfast burrito isn't exactly friendly to those prioritizing their health. This version offers all the deliciousness of a breakfast burrito but with fewer calories and more nutrition.

Olive oil cooking spray

2 medium yellow squash, cut into ½-inch dice

5 sweet mini peppers, thinly sliced

1 medium onion, cut into ¼-inch dice

5 large eggs

1½ cups carton egg whites

2 tablespoons taco seasoning

5 cooked turkey sausage patties, crumbled

2 cups baby spinach

1¼ cups 2% Mexican blend shredded cheese

28 baked tortilla chips, crumbled

Chopped fresh cilantro, for serving (optional)

Hot sauce, for serving (optional)

1. Heat a large nonstick skillet over medium heat. Spray with cooking spray. Add the squash, peppers, and onion and sauté until soft, about 5 minutes.
2. Meanwhile, in a medium bowl, whisk together the eggs, egg whites, and taco seasoning.
3. Add the sausage and spinach to the skillet and cook for 1 to 2 minutes, or until the sausage is heated through and the spinach starts to wilt.
4. Add the eggs to the skillet and combine with the other ingredients. Stir gently every 30 seconds until the eggs are firm and the mixture no longer looks wet, about 10 minutes.

5. Evenly divide the mixture into each of 5 single-compartment prep containers. Top each portion with ¼ cup of cheese, the crumbled tortilla chips, and cilantro and hot sauce (if using). Cover. Store in the refrigerator until needed.

Reheat: From refrigerated, with the lid cracked, heat in the microwave for 1 minute 30 seconds.

Substitution Tip: Experiment with other add-ins such as zucchini, broccoli, or cauliflower. If you want to boost the carbs, use frozen cubed potatoes or sweet potatoes.

Per serving: Calories: 368, Total fat: 20g, Total carbs: 19g, Sugar: 6g, Protein: 30g, Fiber: 3g, Sodium: 922mg

Black Bean Turkey Chili

DAIRY-FREE, GLUTEN-FREE, NUT-FREE, STRENGTH, STRENGTH/CARDIO

PREP TIME: 5 MINUTES / **COOK TIME:** 55 MINUTES • **MAKES 3 SERVINGS**

This is a healthier version of traditional chili con carne, but it doesn't skimp on the chili flavor that people love. The protein comes from lean ground turkey instead of beef, plus a nice dose of plant-based protein from black beans. The spices in chili are strong and can cover the flavor of vegetables really well. Therefore, you can add a powerfully nutritious vegetable boost and not even notice flavor-wise.

1 pound 93% lean ground turkey
1 medium onion, cut into ¼-inch dice
10 baby carrots, grated
1 (28-ounce) can diced tomatoes
2 (15-ounce) cans black beans
2 chili seasoning packets (or 2½ tablespoons chili seasoning)
5 cups coarsely chopped baby spinach

1. Heat a 5-quart pot over medium heat and brown the turkey, stirring and breaking up larger chunks with a spatula, about 15 minutes.
2. Add the onion and carrots and cook for about 5 minutes, or until the onion is soft, stirring frequently.
3. Add the tomatoes, black beans with their juices, chili seasoning, and spinach. Stir until well combined. Continue to cook over medium heat, stirring every couple of minutes, until the mixture comes to a slow boil, about 5 minutes.
4. Cover and reduce the heat to low. Let simmer for about 30 minutes.
5. Turn off the heat, stir, and let cool, uncovered, for 15 minutes.
6. Evenly divide the chili into each of 3 single-compartment prep containers. Cover. Immediately store in the refrigerator until needed.

Reheat: From the refrigerator, with the lid cracked, heat in the microwave for 3 minutes, stirring after each 1-minute increment.

Per serving: Calories: 631, Total fat: 15g, Total carbs: 77g, Sugar: 11g, Protein: 50g, Fiber: 29g, Sodium: 885mg

Lemon Chicken with Quinoa and Spring Greens

DAIRY-FREE, NUT-FREE, POST-WORKOUT, STRENGTH

PREP TIME: 10 MINUTES / **COOK TIME:** 30 MINUTES • **MAKES 2 SERVINGS**

Boneless, skinless chicken breast is a great lean protein choice that has long been recommended by professional bodybuilders and athletes. However, by itself it can be a bit dry, bland, and boring. The lemon and thyme in this recipe permeate the meat, giving it great flavor and helping make chicken breast a much more enjoyable component of your strength-building diet.

1 cup quinoa, rinsed well
2 cups water
3 tablespoons whole wheat flour
½ teaspoon sea salt
½ teaspoon garlic powder
¼ teaspoon freshly ground black pepper
2 tablespoons olive oil, divided
1 pound boneless, skinless chicken breast, halved horizontally to make thin fillets
1 cup chicken broth
Juice of 1½ lemons
½ teaspoon dried thyme
16 cups organic spring salad mix
12 cherry tomatoes
6 sweet mini peppers, thinly sliced
6 baby carrots, thinly sliced

1. In a 2-quart pot over high heat, combine the quinoa and water and bring to a boil. Reduce the heat to low, stir, cover, and cook for about 25 minutes, or until water is fully absorbed.
2. Combine the flour, salt, garlic powder, and black pepper on a plate and mix well.
3. Heat a large nonstick skillet over medium heat with 1 tablespoon of olive oil.
4. Coat the chicken in the flour mixture on both sides and then place in the skillet. Cook for about 5 minutes on one side, or until golden brown, then add the remaining 1 tablespoon of oil, flip the chicken, and brown on the other side for about 5 minutes.
5. Remove the chicken from the skillet and set aside. Add the remaining flour mixture to the skillet and stir with a spoon to dissolve it into the liquid.

>>

Lemon Chicken with Quinoa and Spring Greens continued

6. Add the broth, lemon juice, and thyme and bring to a boil. Return the chicken to the skillet, cover, and reduce the heat to medium-low. Cook for about 8 minutes, then turn the heat off.
7. Evenly divide the spring mix, tomatoes, sweet peppers, and carrots into each of 2 single-compartment prep containers. Cover. Store in the refrigerator until needed.
8. Evenly divide the quinoa, chicken, and sauce into each of 2 separate prep containers. Cover. Store in the refrigerator until needed.

Prep Tip: This salad is designed to store well in the refrigerator for up to 1 week, but if you have time, you can make the salad fresh, right before you're ready to eat.

Reheat: Only the quinoa/chicken will need to be heated. From the refrigerator, with the lid cracked, heat in the microwave for 2 minutes, stirring after each 1-minute increment. Serve on top of the salad.

Per serving: Calories: 887, Total fat: 26g, Total carbs: 98g, Sugar: 16g, Protein: 73g, Fiber: 21g, Sodium: 1,466mg

Albacore Tuna Salad with Whole-Grain Crackers

DAIRY-FREE, NUT-FREE, POST-WORKOUT, STRENGTH, STRENGTH/CARDIO

PREP TIME: 5 MINUTES • **MAKES 5 SERVINGS**

Most people turn to a protein shake after a workout as a way to recover faster and promote muscle growth. However, protein shakes can present problems, especially if you have sensitivities to whey or don't like the texture. This post-workout snack is my go-to protein shake alternative. The protein in tuna is high quality, easy to digest, and readily used by the body. Spend a little more money and choose the "solid white, safe-caught" variety; it tastes better.

2 (12-ounce) cans solid white albacore tuna in water, drained
5 tablespoons light mayonnaise
20 whole-grain crackers

1. In a medium bowl, combine the tuna and mayonnaise and mix well.
2. Evenly divide the tuna salad into each of 5 prep containers. Cover. Place 4 crackers in each of 5 small resealable plastic bags (or small prep containers). Store the tuna salad in the refrigerator until needed. Stir before eating.

Ingredient Tip: You can spread the tuna salad on the crackers or simply crumble the crackers on top and eat with a spoon.

Per serving: Calories: 233, Total fat: 7g, Total carbs: 15g, Sugar: 1g, Protein: 26g, Fiber: 2g, Sodium: 499mg

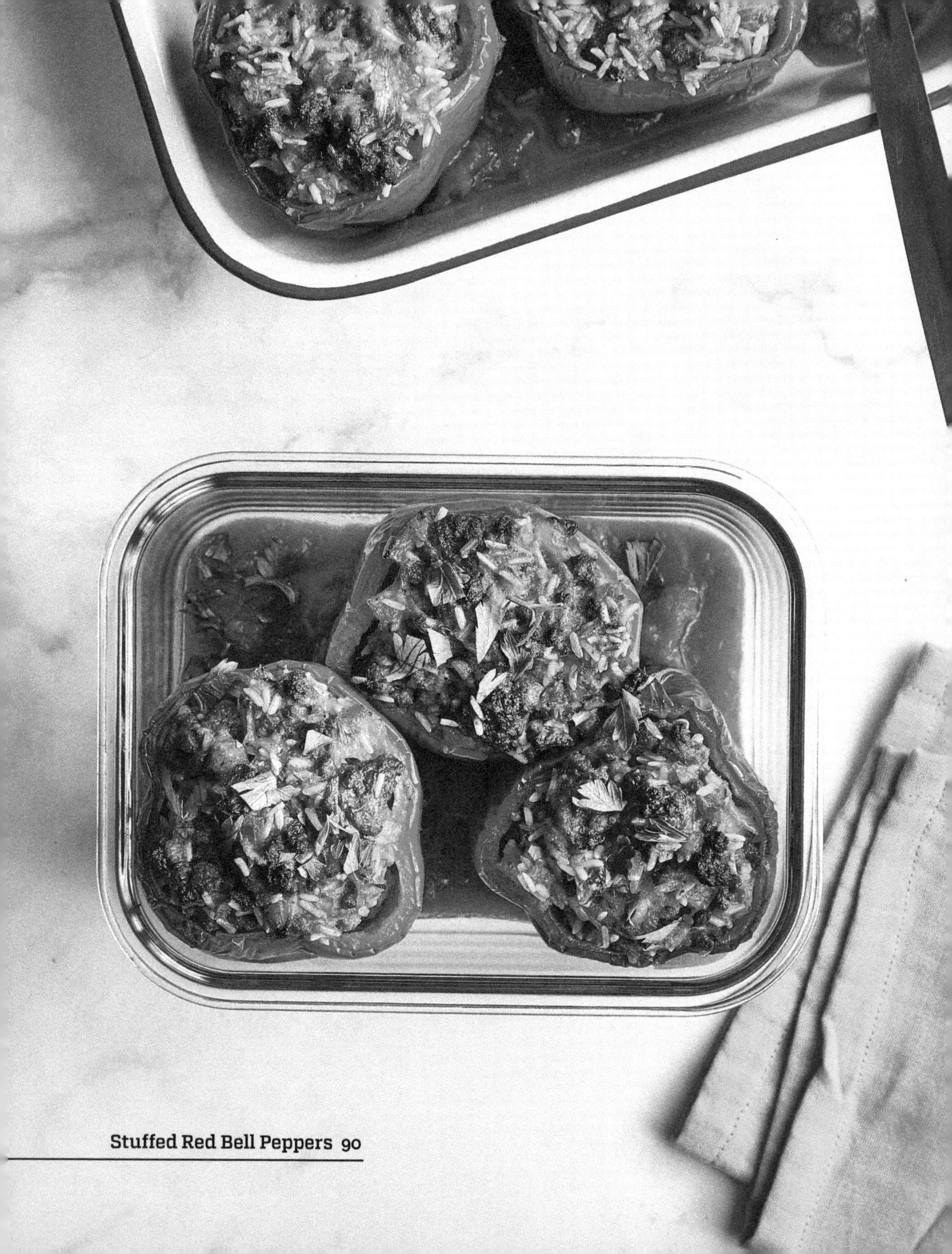

Stuffed Red Bell Peppers 90

CHAPTER FIVE

MEAL PREPS FOR STRENGTH/CARDIO

The following two meal preps are designed to fuel the popular workouts that have both a strength component and a cardio component. As a reminder, the serving sizes were developed for the nutritional needs of a 5'9" 175-pound man doing 45 to 60 minutes of strength/cardio at least four or five times per week, which is the typical length of a cross training–type workout. You may have to adjust the serving sizes, depending on your exact stats and goals (see Calculating Your Daily Macros, page 5, for how to calculate your unique energy needs).

PREP 1

PREP 2

Strength/Cardio Prep 1

This first strength/cardio meal prep has a good balance of whole grains and lean protein. It consists of five easy-to-make meals and some already prepared grab-and-go snacks. You'll start your day with a power bowl, and then your lunches and dinners will be chicken and rice soup, roasted vegetables with chicken, a quinoa harvest bowl, or stuffed bell peppers. Chicken and beef make up the primary protein sources, but this week has a vegetarian option using quinoa.

	BREAKFAST	LUNCH	WORKOUT/ REST	SNACK(S)	DINNER
MONDAY	Blueberry Power Bowl (page 91)	Hearty Chicken and Rice Soup (page 88)	Workout	1 banana, 1 apple, RTD (ready-to-drink) protein shake	Roasted Veggie Bowl with Grilled Chicken (page 89)
TUESDAY	Blueberry Power Bowl	Stuffed Red Bell Peppers (page 90)	Workout	1 banana, 1 apple, RTD protein shake	Quinoa Harvest Bowl with Balsamic Glaze (page 92)
WEDNESDAY	Blueberry Power Bowl	Roasted Veggie Bowl with Grilled Chicken	Rest	1 apple	Hearty Chicken and Rice Soup
THURSDAY	Blueberry Power Bowl	Quinoa Harvest Bowl with Balsamic Glaze	Workout	1 banana, 1 apple, RTD protein shake	Stuffed Red Bell Peppers
FRIDAY	Blueberry Power Bowl	Hearty Chicken and Rice Soup	Workout	1 banana, 1 apple, RTD protein shake	Roasted Veggie Bowl with Grilled Chicken

Prep 1 Shopping List

Pantry

- Balsamic glaze
- Beans, black (1 [15-ounce] can)
- Caesar salad dressing
- Chicken bouillon cubes (3)
- Garlic powder
- Marinara sauce (1 cup)
- Olive oil cooking spray
- Paprika
- Pepper, black
- Sea salt
- Vegetable stock (2 cups)

Produce

- Apples (5)
- Bananas (4)
- Beet (1 large)
- Bell peppers, red (6 large)
- Broccoli florets (4 cups)
- Carrots, baby (1 [16-ounce] bag)
- Cauliflower florets (4 cups)
- Celery (6 stalks)
- Onion, red (1 large)
- Onions, yellow (2 medium)
- Potatoes, yellow (4 medium)
- Spinach, baby (4 cups)
- Sweet mini peppers (10)
- Sweet potatoes (4 medium [4 to 5 inch] or 2 large [7 to 8 inch])

Protein

- Beef, 92% lean grass-fed ground (1 pound)
- Chicken, boneless, skinless breast (2½ pounds)
- Chicken, boneless, skinless thighs (1 pound)

Dairy/Eggs

- Egg (1 large)
- Low-fat vanilla Greek yogurt (5 cups)

Grains

- Quinoa (1 cup)
- Oats, quick-cook rolled (2½ cups)
- Rice, brown (4 cups)

Nuts/Seeds

- Walnuts, chopped (1¼ cups)

Other

- Blueberries, frozen (7½ cups)
- Protein shakes (4 [~30 grams protein each])

Equipment and Storage Vessels

- 2 large baking sheets
- 2-quart pot with lid
- 5-quart pot with lid
- 9-by-13-inch baking pan or casserole dish
- Chef's knife
- Cutting boards (2)
- Fork
- Glass meal prep containers, large single-compartment (12)
- Glass meal prep containers, medium single-compartment (5)
- Large nonstick skillet
- Measuring cups and spoons
- Mixing bowls
- Parchment paper
- Spatula
- Wooden spoons

Step-by-Step Prep

1. Two of the recipes this week incorporate two side dish recipes from chapter 7. Start with these as they can be roasting while you work on the other recipes. Complete all the steps for the Savory Roasted Root Vegetables (page 128) and Roasted Garden Vegetables (page 129). Remember to take the garden vegetables out after 30 minutes and then cook the root vegetables for 20 more minutes.
2. While the vegetables are roasting, complete steps 1 through 3 of the Hearty Chicken and Rice Soup (page 88).
3. While the soup is simmering, use the 2-quart pot to cook the rice in steps 1 and 2 of the Roasted Veggie Bowl with Grilled Chicken (page 89).
4. While the rice cooks, complete steps 1 through 4 of the Stuffed Red Bell Peppers (page 90) to get them ready to put in the oven as soon as the vegetables have finished roasting.
5. While you're waiting for the rice to finish cooking, completely prepare the Blueberry Power Bowl (page 91).
6. When the rice is done, complete steps 3 and 4 of the Roasted Veggie Bowl with Grilled Chicken. Use the 2-quart pot to cook the quinoa in steps 1 and 2 of the Quinoa Harvest Bowl with Balsamic Glaze (page 92).

7. While the quinoa is cooking, complete step 3 of the Roasted Veggie Bowl with Grilled Chicken. Once the chicken is cooked, complete step 5.
8. Next, complete steps 4 and 5 of the Hearty Chicken and Rice Soup.
9. At this stage, your quinoa should be cooked, so complete steps 3 through 5 of the Quinoa Harvest Bowl with Balsamic Glaze.
10. Now finish your meal prep by completing steps 5 through 7 of the Stuffed Red Bell Peppers.

Hearty Chicken and Rice Soup

CARDIO, DAIRY-FREE, GLUTEN-FREE, NUT-FREE, STRENGTH/CARDIO

PREP TIME: 15 MINUTES / **COOK TIME:** 1 HOUR 10 MINUTES • **MAKES 3 SERVINGS**

This super easy, one-pot chicken and rice soup is a hearty way to finish your day or refuel after a good workout. I recently made this for a group of adventure race competitors after their race, and they thought it was the best thing ever. Using boneless, skinless chicken cuts down on the fat that other chicken soups contain, and to compensate for the lack of fat, we add bouillon to boost the flavor.

6 cups water

1 pound boneless, skinless chicken thighs, cut into 1- to 2-inch cubes

1 pound boneless, skinless chicken breast, cut into 1- to 2-inch cubes

1 medium onion, cut into ½-inch dice

6 celery stalks, thinly sliced

4 cups baby spinach

2 cups brown rice, rinsed well

3 chicken bouillon cubes

1 teaspoon freshly ground black pepper

1. In a large 5-quart pot over high heat, bring the water to a boil.
2. Add the chicken, onion, celery, spinach, rice, bouillon cubes, and pepper to the boiling water.
3. Bring the pot back to a boil. Then reduce the heat and simmer for about 50 minutes, stirring a few times while cooking, or until the chicken is cooked through.
4. Remove from the heat and let cool for 20 minutes.
5. Evenly divide the soup into each of 3 large single-compartment prep containers. Cover. Store in the refrigerator until needed.

Ingredient Tip: It may be tempting to skip rinsing the rice, but dried rice contains naturally occurring arsenic. Rinsing the rice for at least a minute removes most of the arsenic.

Reheat: From refrigerated, with the lid cracked, heat in the microwave for 90 seconds, stir, then heat for another minute.

Per serving: Calories: 889, Total fat: 20g, Total carbs: 111g, Sugar: 3g, Protein: 71g, Fiber: 7g, Sodium: 2,548mg

Roasted Veggie Bowl with Grilled Chicken

CARDIO, DAIRY-FREE, GLUTEN-FREE, NUT-FREE, POST-WORKOUT, STRENGTH/CARDIO

PREP TIME: 15 MINUTES / **COOK TIME:** 50 MINUTES • **MAKES 3 SERVINGS**

Roasting vegetables is a great way to enjoy them because they offer a different taste and texture than raw or steamed vegetables. And because roasting retains almost all the vegetables' nutrients, you'll get more micronutrients.

3 cups water

1½ cups brown rice, rinsed well

1½ pounds boneless, skinless chicken breast, cut into 1- to 2-inch cubes

1 teaspoon garlic powder

½ teaspoon sea salt

¼ teaspoon freshly ground black pepper

¼ teaspoon paprika

3 cups Savory Roasted Root Vegetables (page 128)

3 cups Roasted Garden Vegetables (page 129)

6 tablespoons Caesar dressing

1. In a 2-quart pot over high heat, combine the water and rice and bring to a boil.
2. Reduce the heat to low, stir, cover, and cook for about 30 minutes, or until water is fully absorbed.
3. While the rice is cooking, heat a large nonstick skillet over medium heat. In the skillet, combine the chicken, garlic powder, salt, pepper, and paprika. Cook for about 10 minutes, or until the chicken is cooked through.
4. Fluff the rice with a fork. Evenly divide it into each of 3 large single-compartment prep containers.
5. Evenly divide the Savory Roasted Root Vegetables, Roasted Garden Vegetables, and chicken on top of the rice. Drizzle 2 tablespoons of Caesar dressing over each. Cover. Store in the refrigerator until needed.

Prep Tip: Freeze any leftover roasted vegetables for use in other recipes later.

Reheat: From the refrigerator, with the lid cracked, heat in the microwave for 3 minutes, stirring after each 1-minute increment. Add an additional minute if reheating from frozen.

Per serving: Calories: 1,250, Total fat: 37g, Total carbs: 159g, Sugar: 23g, Protein: 70g, Fiber: 18g, Sodium: 2,000mg

Stuffed Red Bell Peppers

DAIRY-FREE, GLUTEN-FREE, NUT-FREE, POST-WORKOUT, STRENGTH/CARDIO, VEGAN OPTION

PREP TIME: 15 MINUTES / **COOK TIME:** 45 MINUTES • **MAKES 2 SERVINGS**

Red bell peppers are high in vitamin C as well as other nutrients, plus they taste great. Here they serve as a "pocket" to hold a rice and beef mixture that's a lower-carb alternative to other pockets, such as tortillas, pita, or rolls.

- **6 large red bell peppers, tops removed, seeds and membranes removed**
- **1 pound 93% lean grass-fed ground beef**
- **½ cup brown rice, rinsed well**
- **1 medium onion, cut into ¼-inch dice**
- **1 teaspoon sea salt**
- **¼ teaspoon freshly ground black pepper**
- **½ teaspoon garlic powder**
- **1 large egg**
- **1 (15-ounce) jar marinara sauce, divided**

1. Preheat the oven to 350°F. Line a 9-by-13-inch baking pan with parchment paper.
2. Arrange the peppers cut-side up in the prepared baking pan.
3. In a medium bowl, combine the beef, rice, onion, salt, black pepper, garlic powder, egg, and ½ cup of marinara sauce. Stir until well combined.
4. Stuff each pepper evenly with the beef mixture. If there's any leftover mixture, simply place in the pan around the peppers. Pour the remaining marinara sauce over the peppers.
5. Place in the oven and bake for about 45 minutes, or until tender.
6. Remove from the oven and let cool for 10 minutes.
7. Place 3 stuffed peppers and half of the sauce from the pan into each of 2 large single-compartment prep containers. Cover. Store in the refrigerator until needed.

Reheat: From the refrigerator, with the lid cracked, heat in the microwave for 3 minutes, stirring after each 1-minute increment. Allow to rest 1 minute before eating.

Substitution Tip: This recipe can be made vegan by swapping the ground beef for two cans of undrained black beans and omitting the egg.

Per serving: Calories: 776, Total fat: 19g, Total carbs: 97g, Sugar: 40g, Protein: 63g, Fiber: 17g, Sodium: 2,106mg

Blueberry Power Bowl

DAIRY-FREE OPTION, GLUTEN-FREE, STRENGTH/CARDIO

PREP TIME: 10 MINUTES • **MAKES 5 SERVINGS**

Blueberries are rich in antioxidants, so if you can make them a regular part of your diet, your body will thank you. This recipe helps you do just that, starting your day with a powerful antioxidant dose, plus healthy carbs from oats, protein from Greek yogurt, and healthy fats from walnuts. Because there's no cooking involved, this recipe is superfast to throw together, even if you can't prep it ahead of time.

7½ cups frozen or fresh blueberries
2½ cups quick-cook rolled oats
5 cups low-fat vanilla Greek yogurt or vanilla plant-based yogurt
1¼ cups chopped walnuts

1. In a medium bowl, combine the blueberries, rolled oats, and yogurt and stir gently until uniform.
2. Evenly divide the mixture into each of 5 medium single-compartment prep containers.
3. Top each with ¼ cup of walnuts. Cover. Store in the refrigerator until needed.

Substitution Tip: Don't like walnuts? You can substitute any nut of your choice.

Per serving: Calories: 710, Total fat: 28g, Total carbs: 91g, Sugar: 46g, Protein: 31g, Fiber: 17g, Sodium: 98mg

Quinoa Harvest Bowl with Balsamic Glaze

CARDIO, GLUTEN-FREE, NUT-FREE, PRE-WORKOUT, STRENGTH/CARDIO, VEGAN

PREP TIME: 15 MINUTES / **COOK TIME:** 50 MINUTES • **MAKES 2 SERVINGS**

Unlike other plant proteins, such as from rice and wheat, quinoa protein is complete. That means it has all the essential amino acids needed by the body. This bowl incorporates two other healthy sides to create a balanced meal.

1 cup quinoa, rinsed well

2 cups vegetable stock

2 cups Savory Roasted Root Vegetables (page 128)

2 cups Roasted Garden Vegetables (page 129)

1 (15-ounce) can black beans, drained

4 tablespoons balsamic glaze, or homemade (see tip)

1. In a 2-quart pot over high heat, combine the quinoa and stock and bring to a boil.
2. Reduce the heat to low, stir, cover, and cook for about 30 minutes, or until liquid is fully absorbed.
3. Remove from the heat and let the quinoa sit for 5 minutes.
4. Fluff the quinoa with a fork and then evenly divide it into each of 2 large single-compartment prep containers.
5. Place 1 cup of Savory Roasted Root Vegetables and 1 cup of Roasted Garden Vegetables in each container on top of the quinoa. Evenly divide the black beans into each container. Drizzle 2 tablespoons of balsamic glaze over each bowl. Cover. Store in the refrigerator until needed.

Ingredient Tip: Making your own balsamic glaze is easy. Simply pour 1 cup balsamic vinegar in a small pot, bring it to a boil, then reduce the heat to simmer for 10 to 15 minutes (or longer, if you want it even thicker).

Reheat: From the refrigerator, with the lid cracked, heat in the microwave for 3 minutes, stirring after each 1-minute increment.

Per serving: Calories: 1,093, Total fat: 18g, Total carbs: 200g, Sugar: 49g, Protein: 33g, Fiber: 38g, Sodium: 1,767mg

Strength/Cardio Prep 2

For this next strength/cardio meal prep, you'll find a few more great protein sources from shrimp and salmon as well as some chicken and beef. You'll also enjoy a flavorful and protein-rich bean salad as your snack each day, which is a great plant-based option. You'll start your day with a generous portion of frittata and then your lunches and dinners will be a rotation of fried rice, beef Burgundy, chicken and bean burritos, and salmon with sweet potato mash. This meal prep is designed to keep your weekly menu interesting and to give you the fuel your body needs for your fitness goals.

	BREAKFAST	LUNCH	WORKOUT/ REST	SNACK(S)	DINNER
MONDAY	Tomato and Cheese Frittata (page 97)	Shrimp Fried Rice (page 99)	Workout	Six-Bean Salad (page 98) and 1 banana or apple	Lean and Savory Beef Burgundy (page 101)
TUESDAY	Tomato and Cheese Frittata	Chicken and Black Bean Burritos (page 103)	Workout	Six-Bean Salad and 1 banana or apple	Panfried Salmon with Sweet Potato Mash (page 105)
WEDNESDAY	Tomato and Cheese Frittata	Lean and Savory Beef Burgundy	Rest	Six-Bean Salad	Shrimp Fried Rice
THURSDAY	Tomato and Cheese Frittata	Chicken and Black Bean Burritos	Workout	Six-Bean Salad and 1 banana or apple	Panfried Salmon with Sweet Potato Mash
FRIDAY	Tomato and Cheese Frittata	Shrimp Fried Rice	Workout	Six-Bean Salad and 1 banana or apple	Lean and Savory Beef Burgundy

Prep 2 Shopping List

Pantry

- Apple cider vinegar
- Basil, dried
- Bay leaves
- Beans, black (2 [15-ounce] cans)
- Beans, green (1 [15-ounce] can)
- Beans, kidney (1 [15-ounce] can)
- Beans, lima beans (1 [15-ounce] can)
- Beans, white (1 [15-ounce] can)
- Beef broth (2 cups)
- Bread crumbs, Italian-style (1 cup)
- Chickpeas (1 [15-ounce] can)
- Dill, dried
- Garlic powder
- Ginger, ground
- Oil, coconut
- Oil, olive
- Olive oil cooking spray
- Paprika
- Pepper, black
- Salsa, prepared (8 tablespoons)
- Sea salt
- Soy sauce, reduced-sodium
- Sugar, brown
- Taco seasoning
- Tomato paste
- Thyme, dried
- Wine, red (inexpensive) (2 cups)

Produce

- Apples or bananas (4)
- Bell pepper, green (1)
- Broccoli florets (5 cups)
- Carrots, baby (1 [16-ounce] bag)
- Lemon (1)
- Mushrooms, presliced white button (4 cups)
- Onions, yellow (2 medium)
- Onion, sweet (1 medium)
- Potatoes, yellow (6 medium)
- Spinach, baby (9 cups)
- Sweet potatoes (4 medium [5 inch] or 2 large [7 to 8 inch])
- Tomatoes, cherry (15)

Protein

- Beef, lean (sirloin or similar) (1½ pounds)
- Chicken, boneless, skinless breast (8 ounces)
- Salmon, fresh (2 [5-ounce] fillets)
- Shrimp, frozen, peeled, deveined, tail-off, precooked (1 pound)

Dairy

- 2% milk or milk alternative (1 cup)
- Egg whites, carton (2½ cups)
- Eggs (9 large)
- Feta cheese crumbles (6 ounces)

Grains

- Bread, whole-grain (5 slices)
- Rice, brown (2½ cups)
- Tortillas, low-carb burrito size (4)

Other

- Onions, frozen, small pearl (1 small bag)
- Peas, frozen (2 cups)

Equipment and Storage Vessels

- 2-quart pot with lid
- 5-quart pot with lid
- 9-by-13-inch baking pan
- Chef's knife
- Cutting boards (2)
- Fork
- Glass meal prep containers, double-compartment (2)
- Glass meal prep containers, large single-compartment (8)
- Glass meal prep containers, medium single-compartment (10)
- Large cast-iron skillet
- Large nonstick skillet
- Measuring cups and spoons
- Mixing bowls
- Parchment paper
- Potato masher (optional)
- Small saucepan
- Spatula
- Whisk
- Wooden spoons

Step-by-Step Prep

1. Start your meal prep this week by completing steps 1 through 4 of the Lean and Savory Beef Burgundy (page 101) as this takes the longest to cook.
2. Once that recipe is simmering, complete steps 1 and 2 to cook the brown rice for the Shrimp Fried Rice (page 99) and step 1 to cook the brown rice for the Chicken and Black Bean Burritos (page 103).
3. While the rice is cooking, complete steps 1 through 3 of the Tomato and Cheese Frittata (page 97).
4. Next, use a cast-iron skillet to complete steps 3 and 4 of the Shrimp Fried Rice. When that is finished cooking, the rice should now be ready to add (step 5). Reserve 2 cups of cooked rice for the burritos. Complete steps 6 through 8 of the Shrimp Fried Rice.

5. Complete steps 5 and 6 of the Tomato and Cheese Frittata, and then complete steps 2 through 6 of the Chicken and Black Bean Burritos.
6. Using the microwave and a nonstick skillet, complete all steps for the Pan-fried Salmon with Sweet Potato Mash (page 105).
7. Check on the Lean and Savory Beef Burgundy, as it may be time to complete step 5.
8. While that is cooking its last 20 minutes, complete all steps for the Six-Bean Salad (page 98).
9. Once the Lean and Savory Beef Burgundy has finished cooking, complete steps 6 and 7.

Tomato and Cheese Frittata

NUT-FREE, STRENGTH/CARDIO, VEGETARIAN

PREP TIME: 15 MINUTES / **COOK TIME:** 25 MINUTES • **MAKES 5 SERVINGS**

This recipe is a great way to make breakfasts for an entire week or breakfast for your friends and family. The protein content is boosted using egg whites instead of all whole eggs, which cuts down on the fat and cholesterol. There are no rules when it comes to what you can put in a frittata, so use this recipe as a base and experiment with your own add-ins in the weeks to come.

5 large eggs
2½ cups carton egg whites
½ cup milk or milk alternative
5 slices whole-grain bread, cut into 1-inch cubes
15 cherry tomatoes, halved
5 cups coarsely chopped baby spinach
2 cups coarsely chopped broccoli florets
6 ounces feta cheese crumbles
1 teaspoon sea salt
¼ teaspoon freshly ground black pepper

1. Preheat the oven to 350°F. Line a 9-by-13-inch baking pan with parchment paper.
2. In a medium bowl, combine the eggs, egg whites, and milk and whisk until combined and fluffy, 1 to 2 minutes.
3. Add the bread, tomatoes, spinach, broccoli, feta, salt, and pepper and mix with a spoon until well combined.
4. Pour the mixture into the prepared baking pan and place in the oven on the middle rack. Cook for about 25 minutes, or until the middle is no longer glossy and jiggly.
5. Remove from the oven and let cool 15 minutes.
6. Evenly divide the finished frittata into each of 5 medium meal single-compartment prep containers. Cover. Store in the refrigerator until needed.

Reheat: From the refrigerator, with the lid cracked, heat in the microwave for 60 to 90 seconds. Check after 1 minute and heat an additional 30 seconds if needed.

Per serving: Calories: 383, Total fat: 15g, Total carbs: 30g, Sugar: 10g, Protein: 32g, Fiber: 7g, Sodium: 1,335mg

Six-Bean Salad

GLUTEN-FREE, NUT-FREE, PRE-WORKOUT, STRENGTH/CARDIO, VEGAN

PREP TIME: 15 MINUTES / **COOK TIME:** 5 MINUTES • **MAKES 5 SERVINGS**

This bean salad is a tasty way to get a lot of plant-based protein as well as healthy carbs to fuel your workouts. This is a marinated-type recipe, designed to sit in the refrigerator and absorb all the flavors and spices, so it's perfect for meal prep. There are many different kinds of beans, so experiment to find the combination you like best. The beans used here are a framework to get you started.

1 (15-ounce) can black beans, drained
1 (15-ounce) can white beans, drained
1 (15-ounce) can kidney beans, drained
1 (15-ounce) can lima beans, drained
1 (15-ounce) can green beans, drained
1 (15-ounce) can chickpeas, drained
1 green bell pepper, cut into ¼-inch dice
1 medium sweet onion, cut into ¼-inch dice
¾ cup apple cider vinegar
½ cup packed brown sugar (or agave or coconut sugar)
½ cup olive oil
½ teaspoon sea salt
¼ teaspoon freshly ground black pepper
¼ teaspoon paprika
½ teaspoon dried dill
½ teaspoon dried basil

1. In a medium bowl, combine the black beans, white beans, kidney beans, lima beans, green beans, chickpeas, bell pepper, and onion.
2. In a small saucepan over medium heat, combine the vinegar, brown sugar, oil, salt, pepper, paprika, dill, and basil and cook until the sugar is dissolved, about 5 minutes.
3. Pour the liquid over the bean mixture and stir gently until the beans are fully coated.
4. Evenly divide the bean salad into each of 5 medium single-compartment prep containers. Cover. Store in the refrigerator until needed. (The bean salad should marinate for at least 1 to 2 hours before eating.)

Substitution Tip: If you don't like onion or green pepper, feel free to omit them. You could use cucumber or celery instead.

Per serving: Calories: 686, Total fat: 25g, Total carbs: 93g, Sugar: 24g, Protein: 25g, Fiber: 27g, Sodium: 249mg

Shrimp Fried Rice

DAIRY-FREE, STRENGTH/CARDIO, VEGAN OPTION

PREP TIME: 15 MINUTES / **COOK TIME:** 40 MINUTES • **MAKES 3 SERVINGS**

This Chinese-inspired meal is a great way to incorporate lean protein, complex carbs, and vegetables into your fitness-oriented diet. It combines several flavors and textures to keep things interesting. If you aren't a fan of shrimp, you can easily use chicken or lean beef instead. This is a much healthier version of fried rice than you might typically find in restaurants.

3 cups water
1½ cups brown rice, rinsed well
1 tablespoon coconut oil
1 medium onion, chopped
15 baby carrots, sliced
3 cups coarsely chopped broccoli
2 cups frozen green peas
2 cups thinly sliced white button mushrooms
1 teaspoon garlic powder
¼ teaspoon ground ginger
¼ teaspoon freshly ground black pepper
½ cup reduced-sodium soy sauce
3 large eggs
1 pound frozen peeled, deveined, and tail-off precooked shrimp

1. In a 2-quart pot over high heat, combine the water and rice and bring to a full boil, stirring occasionally.
2. Reduce the heat to low, stir, and cover. Cook for about 30 minutes, or until water is fully absorbed.
3. In a large cast-iron skillet over medium-high heat, heat the oil. Add the onion, carrots, and broccoli and stir-fry for about 5 minutes, or until the vegetables are as soft as you prefer.
4. Add the peas and mushrooms and stir-fry for about another 5 minutes, or until the peas are heated through.
5. Add the garlic powder, ginger, pepper, and soy sauce, then stir in the cooked rice.
6. Crack the eggs over different sections of the skillet and stir slowly to cook the eggs without mixing them in completely, about 3 minutes.

>>

Shrimp Fried Rice continued

7. Add the shrimp and continue stirring every 30 seconds or so until the shrimp are thawed and hot, about 5 minutes.
8. Remove from the heat. Immediately evenly divide the mixture into each of 3 large single-compartment meal prep containers. Cover. Store in the refrigerator until needed.

Reheat: From the refrigerator, with the lid cracked, heat in the microwave for 3 minutes, stirring gently after each 1-minute increment.

Substitution Tip: Make this vegan by omitting the egg and swapping out the shrimp for two (15-ounce) cans of fava beans.

Per serving: Calories: 760, Total fat: 13g, Total carbs: 106g, Sugar: 12g, Protein: 57g, Fiber: 13g, Sodium: 2,210mg

Lean and Savory Beef Burgundy

DAIRY-FREE, GLUTEN-FREE, NUT-FREE, STRENGTH/CARDIO

PREP TIME: 15 MINUTES / **COOK TIME:** 2 HOURS • **MAKES 3 SERVINGS**

This is the French-inspired version of beef stew. What makes it "French inspired"? The red wine, of course. Red wine adds a layer of flavor that traditional beef stew doesn't have, making for a complex, savory experience. French cooking isn't known for being easy, but I've simplified this recipe so it won't take all day to make and will be a great meal to enjoy to recover from your workouts.

1 tablespoon olive oil

1½ pounds lean beef (sirloin or similar lean cut), cut into 1- to 2-inch cubes

1 medium onion, chopped into ½-inch pieces

2 cups beef broth

2 cups red wine

15 baby carrots

6 medium yellow potatoes, cut into 1- to 2-inch cubes

1 tablespoon garlic powder

¼ teaspoon freshly ground black pepper

2 bay leaves

2 tablespoons tomato paste

1 teaspoon dried thyme

2 cups sliced mushrooms

12 frozen pearl onions

1 teaspoon sea salt

1. In a 5-quart pot, heat the oil over medium heat. Add the beef and cook until browned, stirring every few seconds, about 5 minutes.
2. Add the onion and cook an additional 3 minutes, stirring every few seconds.
3. Add the broth, wine, carrots, potatoes, garlic powder, pepper, bay leaves, tomato paste, and thyme. Increase the heat to medium-high and bring to a boil.
4. Cover, reduce the heat to low, and simmer for about 90 minutes, until the beef is tender.
5. Add the mushrooms, pearl onions, and salt. Cover and simmer for about another 20 minutes, or until the pearl onions are warmed through.

>>

Lean and Savory Beef Burgundy continued

6. Turn off the heat and let rest/cool for 15 minutes. Remove the bay leaves.
7. Evenly divide the mixture into each of 3 large single-compartment prep containers. Cover. Store in the refrigerator until needed.

Reheat: From the refrigerator, with the lid cracked, heat in the microwave for 3 minutes, stirring after each 1-minute increment.

Per serving: Calories: 896, Total fat: 16g, Total carbs: 96g, Sugar: 12g, Protein: 64g, Fiber: 11g, Sodium: 1,655mg

Chicken and Black Bean Burritos

DAIRY-FREE, NUT-FREE, STRENGTH/CARDIO

PREP TIME: 10 MINUTES / COOK TIME: 35 MINUTES • MAKES 2 SERVINGS

Tortillas are pretty high in carbs/calories, so they can scare a lot of fitness-inclined people away. Luckily, there are now several brands of low-carb tortillas. A few years ago, when they first showed up on shelves, I wasn't too impressed. However, they've come a long way. Now you can find great low-carb tortillas that taste just like the real thing, which makes them perfect for lower-carb burritos.

1 cup brown rice, rinsed well
2 cups water
Olive oil cooking spray
8 ounces boneless, skinless chicken breast, cut into 1-inch cubes
1 medium onion, cut into ¼-inch dice
2 tablespoons taco seasoning
4 burrito-size low-carb tortillas
1 (15-ounce) can black beans, drained
8 tablespoons prepared salsa
4 cups baby spinach

1. In a 2-quart pot, combine the rice and water. Bring to a boil over high heat, then turn the heat to low, stir, cover, and simmer for about 30 minutes, or until water is fully absorbed.
2. While the rice cooks, heat a large nonstick skillet over medium heat and spray with cooking spray.
3. Add the chicken, onion, and taco seasoning and cook for about 10 minutes, or until the chicken is fully cooked, stirring regularly. Turn off the heat and let rest.
4. When the rice is done, assemble the burritos. Place 1 tortilla on a plate. Add ½ cup of rice, one-fourth of the chicken mixture, one-fourth of the beans, 2 tablespoons of salsa, and 1 cup of spinach.
5. Fold in the sides of the tortilla and then roll it toward you. Repeat to make the remaining 3 burritos.

>>

Chicken and Black Bean Burritos continued

6. Place 2 burritos in each of 2 large single-compartment storage containers. Cover. Store in the refrigerator until needed.

Ingredient Tip: My favorite brand of low-carb tortilla is La Banderita; it has great taste and texture.

Reheat: From the refrigerator, wrap each burrito in a moist paper towel, put both back in the container, and replace the lid but crack it slightly. Heat for 2 minutes. Allow to rest 1 minute before eating.

Per serving: Calories: 997, Total fat: 14g, Total carbs: 178g, Sugar: 9g, Protein: 63g, Fiber: 50g, Sodium: 1,936mg

Panfried Salmon with Sweet Potato Mash

NUT-FREE, POST-WORKOUT, STRENGTH/CARDIO

PREP TIME: 15 MINUTES / **COOK TIME:** 30 MINUTES • **MAKES 2 SERVINGS**

Salmon is a great protein source for muscle recovery because it contains not only high-quality protein but also anti-inflammatory omega-3 fatty acids. Pairing it with a healthy carb source like sweet potatoes makes for a meal designed to refuel and recharge. Salmon is a flavorful fish, so if it's too much for you, make this recipe with a mild white fish such as tilapia or cod.

4 medium (5-inch) red sweet potatoes
1 teaspoon sea salt (divided)
½ cup 2% milk or milk alternative
¼ teaspoon freshly ground black pepper
2 (5-ounce) fresh salmon fillets
1 large egg
1 cup Italian-style bread crumbs
½ teaspoon garlic powder
½ teaspoon paprika
Olive oil cooking spray
1 lemon, halved lengthwise, for serving (optional)

1. Wash the sweet potatoes and puncture them with a fork on all sides.
2. Cook the sweet potatoes on a paper towel in the microwave for 5 minutes. Turn over each sweet potato and cook for 4 more minutes.
3. Cover with a bowl and let rest for 5 minutes.
4. Cut each potato in half and scoop out all the flesh into a medium bowl. Mash using a fork or potato masher.
5. Add ½ teaspoon of the salt, the milk, and pepper and stir until smooth and creamy.
6. While the sweet potatoes are cooking, rinse and pat dry the salmon with a paper towel.
7. In a shallow bowl, beat the egg. In another shallow bowl, mix together the bread crumbs, garlic powder, the remaining ½ teaspoon of salt, and the paprika.

>>

Panfried Salmon with Sweet Potato Mash continued

8. Spray a large nonstick skillet with cooking spray and preheat over medium heat.
9. Dip each salmon fillet in the egg and then coat with the bread crumb mixture on both sides. Press the crumbs onto the fish with your fingers for a thicker coating.
10. Place the fillets in the skillet and cook for about 7 minutes, then flip with a spatula and cook for about 7 more minutes, until no longer translucent.
11. Remove from the heat and let rest for 5 minutes.
12. Place half the sweet potato mash, a lemon half (if using), and 1 salmon fillet in each of 2 double-compartment meal prep containers. Cover. Store in the refrigerator until needed.

Reheat: From the refrigerator, with the lid off, heat in the microwave for 3 minutes, checking after each 1-minute increment. If desired, squeeze lemon over the salmon before eating.

Per serving: Calories: 676, Total fat: 11g, Total carbs: 95g, Sugar: 21g, Protein: 45g, Fiber: 12g, Sodium: 2,402mg

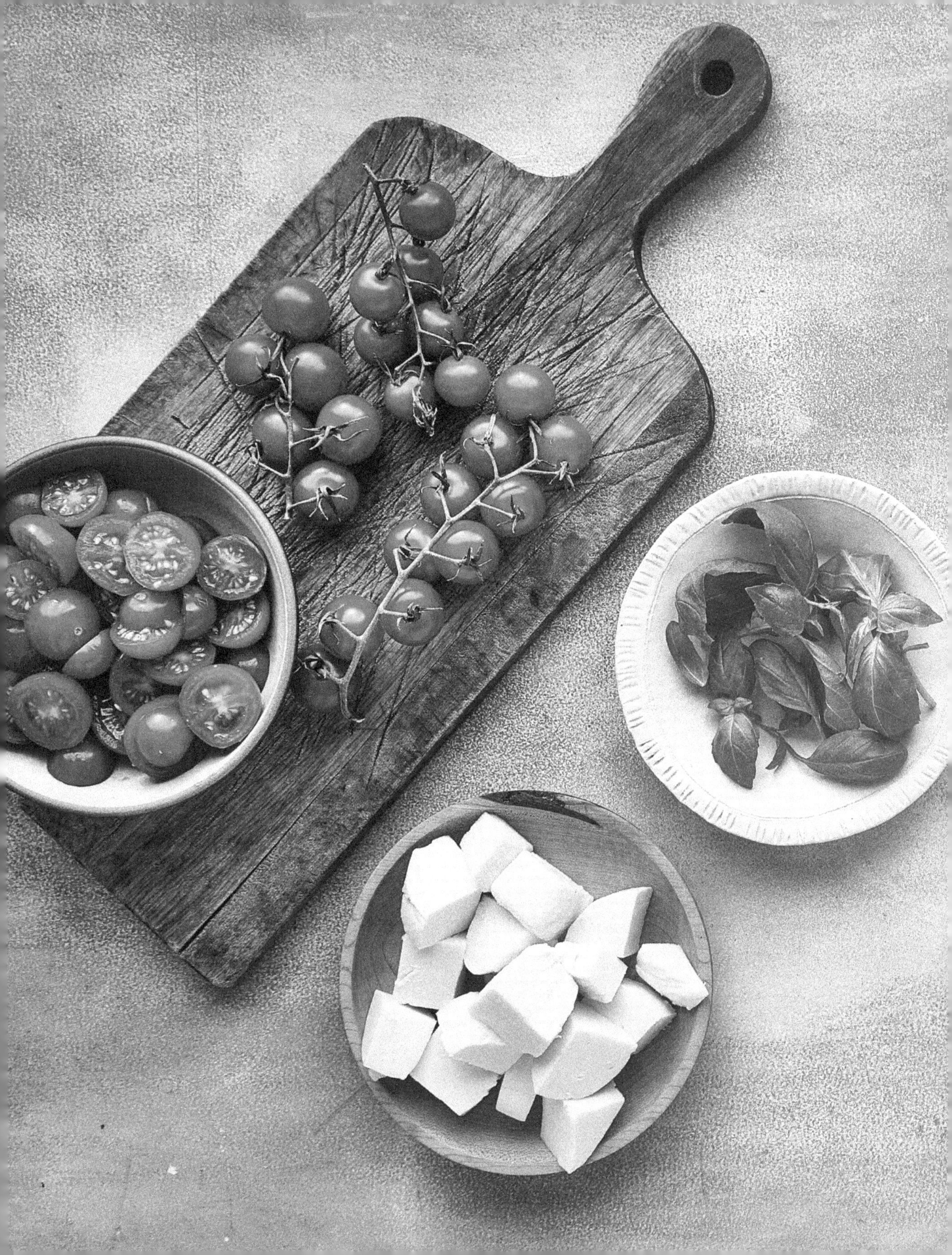

PART THREE

MORE RECIPES TO PREP

Now that you have a feel for how meal prep works and have some basic preps under your belt, here are 42 more recipes that you can use to design your own weekly meal preps to keep your diet interesting and keep moving toward your fitness goals. The following recipes are divided into four categories: Hearty Breakfasts and Smoothies, Power Snacks and Sides, Mighty Mains, and Something Sweet. Pay attention to the recipe labels and use them according to how they fit with your exercise type, goals, and nutritional needs.

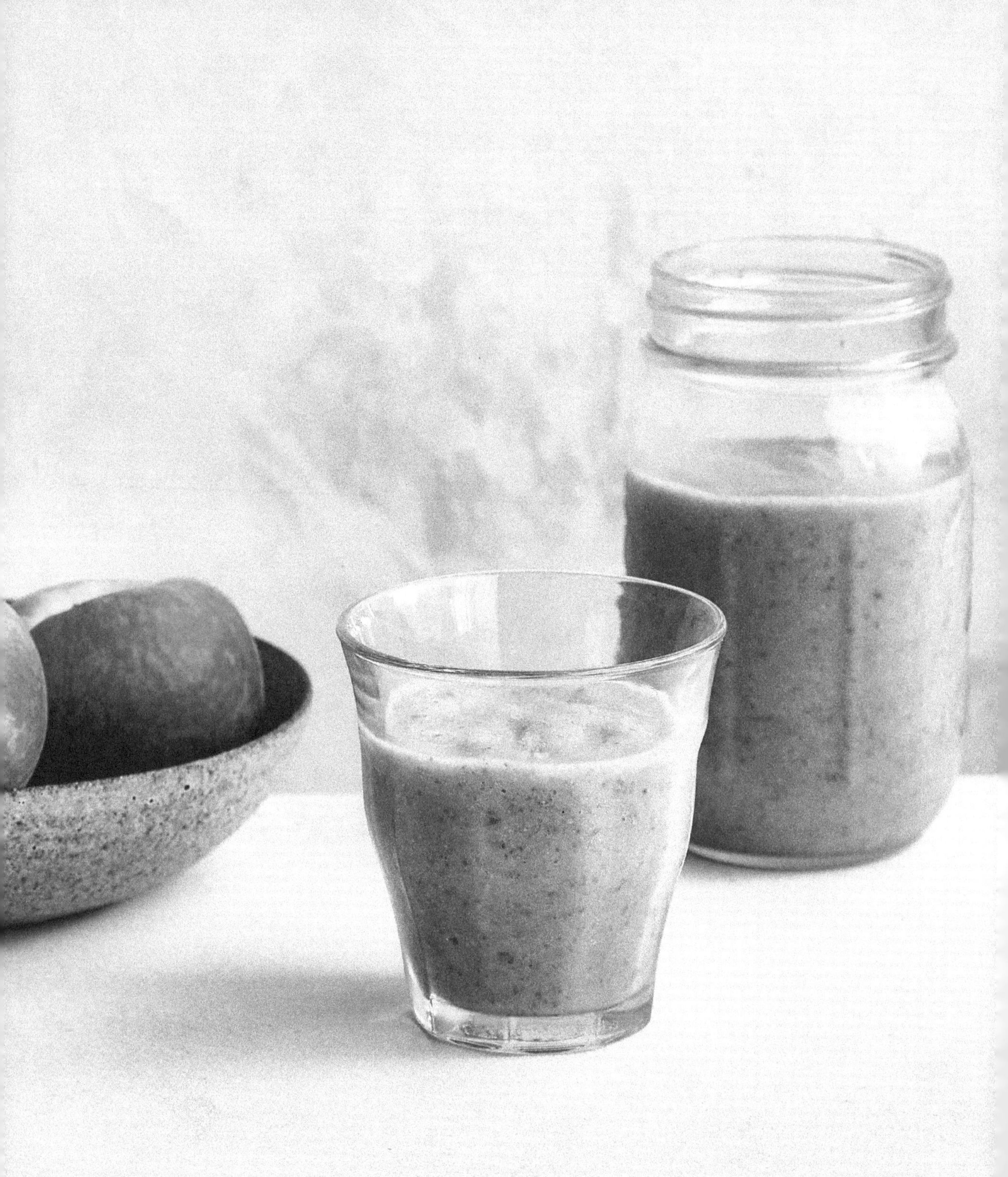

Peach and Chia Smoothie 123

CHAPTER SIX

HEARTY BREAKFASTS AND SMOOTHIES

Apple Cinnamon Overnight Steel-Cut Oats

CARDIO, GLUTEN-FREE, VEGETARIAN

PREP TIME: 15 MINUTES • **MAKES 5 SERVINGS**

Overnight oats are an easy way to enjoy the nutritional benefits of oats without any cooking involved. Let time do the work instead of you. The combinations are endless, so use this recipe as a guide and don't be afraid to get creative with your own mix-ins.

2½ cups water

2 cups 2% milk or plant-based alternative

2½ cups quick-cook steel-cut oats

5 tablespoons honey

2 teaspoons ground cinnamon

1 cup ¼-inch diced dried apples

1 cup coarsely chopped pecans

1. Evenly divide the water and milk into each of 5 prep containers.
2. Add ½ cup of oats to each container and stir.
3. Stir 1 tablespoon of honey into each container.
4. Top each container evenly with the cinnamon, apples, and pecans.
5. Cover. Store in the refrigerator. Allow to rest in the refrigerator overnight for best results.

Reheat: This recipe can be eaten cold or warm. If you want it warm, crack the lid and heat in the microwave for 90 seconds.

Per serving: Calories: 588, Total fat: 23g, Total carbs: 97g, Sugar: 34g, Protein: 14g, Fiber: 12g, Sodium: 67mg

Ham and Cheese Breakfast Bites

NUT-FREE, STRENGTH

PREP TIME: 10 MINUTES / **COOK TIME:** 30 MINUTES • **MAKES 5 SERVINGS**

Ham and cheese is a great flavor combination. By making a few smart ingredient choices, those flavors can be part of a healthy breakfast. Egg whites boost the protein content without adding fat and cholesterol, and the spinach and mini peppers boost the micronutrient content. When choosing ham and other deli meats, always choose uncured varieties, because nitrates aren't great for your health.

5 large eggs

2½ cups carton egg whites

½ cup milk or plant-based alternative

5 slices whole-grain bread, cut into 1-inch cubes

6 ounces uncured Canadian bacon, cut into ½-inch dice

1 medium onion, cut into ¼-inch dice

3 cups coarsely chopped baby spinach

5 sweet mini peppers, cut into ¼-inch dice

1 teaspoon sea salt

¼ teaspoon freshly ground black pepper

1 cup 2% shredded sharp cheddar cheese

Olive oil cooking spray

1. Preheat the oven to 350°F.
2. In a medium bowl, whisk together the eggs, egg whites, and milk.
3. Stir in the bread cubes, Canadian bacon, onion, spinach, sweet peppers, salt, black pepper, and cheese until the mixture is uniform and the bread looks wet.
4. Spray the insides of 10 wells of a nonstick muffin pan with cooking spray. Evenly divide the egg mixture into each of the 10 wells.
5. Place in the oven on the middle rack and bake for about 30 minutes, or until a toothpick comes out clean when stuck into the center of an egg bite.
6. Remove from the oven and allow to cool for 10 to 15 minutes.

>>

Ham and Cheese Breakfast Bites continued

7. Place 2 egg bites in each of 5 meal prep containers. Cover. Store in the refrigerator or freezer until needed.

Reheat: From refrigerated, with the lid cracked, heat in the microwave for 45 seconds. Allow to rest another 45 seconds before eating. From frozen, wrap 2 bites in a moist paper towel and heat in the microwave on 50 percent power for 1 minute. Heat for an additional 1 minute on high power.

Per serving (1 bite): Calories: 400, Total fat: 13g, Total carbs: 29g, Sugar: 9g, Protein: 38g, Fiber: 6g, Sodium: 1,430mg

Avocado on Whole-Grain Toast

CARDIO, NUT-FREE, PRE-WORKOUT, VEGAN

PREP TIME: 5 MINUTES / **COOK TIME:** 5 MINUTES • **MAKES 1 SERVING**

Avocado toast is a superfast breakfast option that offers a good balance of complex carbs and healthy fats to keep you feeling satisfied during your morning. This recipe serves as the basic version, and I've included some other possible add-ons in the tip.

2 slices whole-grain bread
1 medium ripe avocado
Sea salt
Freshly ground black pepper

1. Toast the bread for 3 to 4 minutes.
2. Cut the avocado in half, remove the seed, and cut the avocado flesh in a criss-cross fashion.
3. When the toast is ready, use a spoon to scrape out half the avocado onto each slice of toast and spread evenly.
4. Add salt and pepper to taste and any other toppings you like.
5. This can be placed in a prep container and taken with you. The avocado will last an hour or two before turning brown.

Ingredient Tip: Use frozen, thawed avocado chunks portioned into containers for greater ease of meal prep.

Substitution Tip: Try adding any one or combination of these toppings to liven things up: hot sauce, smoked salmon, cooked bacon, fresh tomato, hard-boiled egg, pumpkin seeds, cilantro, baby spinach, prosciutto, bean sprouts, black beans, lime juice, or garlic powder.

Per serving: Calories: 467, Total fat: 25g, Total carbs: 56g, Sugar: 10g, Protein: 13g, Fiber: 19g, Sodium: 371mg

Hearty Breakfast Sandwich

NUT-FREE, STRENGTH, STRENGTH/CARDIO

PREP TIME: 10 MINUTES / **COOK TIME:** 10 MINUTES • **MAKES 6 SERVINGS**

Breakfast sandwiches are a popular quick breakfast option at fast-food restaurants and coffeehouses. Here's how you can make your own that is not only healthier but a lot more affordable.

6 large eggs
1 cup carton egg whites
½ teaspoon sea salt
¼ teaspoon freshly ground black pepper
Olive oil cooking spray
6 cooked turkey sausage patties
6 slices sharp cheddar cheese
6 whole-grain English muffins, toasted

1. In a medium bowl, whisk together the eggs, egg whites, salt, and pepper.
2. Spray a large nonstick skillet with cooking spray and heat over medium-low heat. Add the eggs, cover, and cook for 8 to 10 minutes, or until done. Remove from the heat and use a spatula to divide the eggs equally into 6 wedges.
3. Assemble the sandwiches by placing an egg wedge, a sausage patty, and a slice of cheese between the halves of each English muffin.
4. For use during the week, place in a prep container and cover. For use beyond that, wrap the sandwich in plastic wrap and freeze.

Reheat: From the refrigerator, wrap the sandwich in a moist paper towel and heat for 1 minute in the microwave. From frozen, remove the plastic wrap, wrap in a moist paper towel, and heat for 2 minutes on 50 percent power and then 1 minute on full power.

Per serving (1 sandwich): Calories: 399, Total fat: 20g, Total carbs: 28g, Sugar: 7g, Protein: 29g, Fiber: 4g, Sodium: 954mg

Protein Pancakes

CARDIO, NUT-FREE, STRENGTH/CARDIO, VEGETARIAN

PREP TIME: 5 MINUTES / **COOK TIME:** 15 MINUTES • **MAKES 4 SERVINGS**

The problem with most protein pancakes is that they can be too dense or too dry. This recipe solves that problem by adding a secret ingredient—applesauce. A little applesauce keeps the pancakes moist, and being conservative with the protein powder keeps them light and fluffy.

2 cups whole wheat flour
2 teaspoons baking powder
2 scoops vanilla protein powder
½ teaspoon sea salt
3 large eggs
½ cup applesauce
1 tablespoon light olive oil
2 cups water

1. In a medium bowl, combine the flour, baking powder, protein powder, and salt. Add the eggs, applesauce, oil, and water and mix until just combined. (It's okay if there are a few lumps; overmixing causes chewy pancakes.)
2. Heat a large nonstick skillet or griddle over medium heat.
3. Pour ½ cup of the batter at a time into the skillet. Flip the pancake when the edges start to appear done, 1 to 2 minutes per side. Don't overcook, as this will dry them out.
4. Repeat until all the batter is used. You should have enough to make 8 pancakes.
5. Any pancakes not eaten immediately can be placed in a prep container and stored in the refrigerator until needed.

Reheat: Wrap 2 pancakes in a moist paper towel and heat in the microwave for 30 to 45 seconds.

Per serving (2 pancakes): Calories: 379, Total fat: 10g, Total carbs: 52g, Sugar: 6g, Protein: 25g, Fiber: 7g, Sodium: 660mg

Scrambled Eggs with Yellow Squash

DAIRY-FREE, GLUTEN-FREE, NUT-FREE, STRENGTH, STRENGTH/CARDIO, VEGETARIAN

PREP TIME: 10 MINUTES / **COOK TIME:** 15 MINUTES • **MAKES 5 SERVINGS**

Mixing yellow squash into scrambled eggs boosts the nutrition and is a lower-calorie alternative to hash browns or other potatoes. The squash also adds bulk, which makes the meal feel more filling. Yellow squash is high in a bunch of vitamins and minerals, so eat plenty.

Olive oil cooking spray
3 medium yellow squash, cut into ½-inch dice
1 medium onion, cut into ¼-inch dice
4 cups baby spinach
1 teaspoon sea salt
¼ teaspoon freshly ground black pepper
5 large eggs
2 cups carton egg whites

1. Spray a large nonstick skillet with cooking spray and heat over medium heat.
2. Add the squash, onion, spinach, salt, and pepper and gently sauté for about 10 minutes, or until the squash and onion are soft.
3. Add the eggs and egg whites and scramble them into the squash mixture. Keep scrambling every 30 seconds for about 5 minutes, or until the eggs are firm.
4. Remove from the heat and evenly divide into each of 5 medium single-compartment prep containers. Cover. Store in the refrigerator until needed.

Reheat: From the refrigerator, with the lid cracked, heat in the microwave for 90 seconds.

Per serving: Calories: 165, Total fat: 6g, Total carbs: 7g, Sugar: 5g, Protein: 19g, Fiber: 2g, Sodium: 719mg

Blueberry Banana Breakfast Muffins

CARDIO, NUT-FREE, VEGAN

PREP TIME: 15 MINUTES / **COOK TIME:** 25 MINUTES • **MAKES 12 MUFFINS**

A sweet pastry tastes great with morning coffee, but most pastries aren't exactly a good fit with a fitness-oriented diet. However, I've adapted this recipe to be both healthy and delicious, so go ahead and enjoy.

1½ cups whole wheat pastry flour
1 teaspoon baking powder
1 teaspoon baking soda
½ teaspoon sea salt
½ cup packed brown sugar
1 medium ripe avocado, mashed
1 ripe banana, mashed
½ cup plant-based milk
⅓ cup olive oil
1 teaspoon vanilla extract
Olive oil cooking spray
1 cup frozen or fresh blueberries

1. Preheat the oven to 350°F.
2. In a medium bowl, stir together the flour, baking powder, baking soda, and salt.
3. In a blender, combine the brown sugar, avocado, banana, plant-based milk, oil, and vanilla and blend until smooth.
4. Add the wet ingredients to the dry ingredients, being sure to scape everything out of the blender cup with a rubber scraper, and mix until just combined. (It's okay if it's a little lumpy.)
5. Spray the insides of a 12-well nonstick muffin pan with cooking spray. Evenly divide the muffin batter into each of the 12 wells.
6. Divide the blueberries between the tops of the muffins, pressing them lightly into the batter.
7. Bake for 25 minutes, or until a toothpick comes out clean when stuck into the center of a muffin.
8. Allow to cool for 10 to 15 minutes before removing from the muffin pan.

>>

9. These will stay fresh for a few days in a sealed container at room temperature. They can also be wrapped individually and frozen.

Reheat: From the refrigerator, heat in the microwave for 10 to 15 seconds. From the freezer, heat the wrapped muffin for 45 seconds in the microwave.

Substitution Tip: If you can't find whole wheat pastry flour, regular whole wheat flour or all-purpose unbleached flour will work, too, as will gluten-free baking flour blends.

Per serving (2 muffins): Calories: 341, Total fat: 16g, Total carbs: 47g, Sugar: 18g, Protein: 4g, Fiber: 7g, Sodium: 504mg

Sunrise Egg and Sausage Skillet

GLUTEN-FREE, NUT-FREE, STRENGTH, STRENGTH/CARDIO

PREP TIME: 10 MINUTES / **COOK TIME:** 25 MINUTES • **MAKES 5 SERVINGS**

This breakfast recipe combines all the great morning flavors people love in one easy-to-make recipe. It stores well so you can start your days with a good balance of protein and healthy carbs. There are a lot of vegetable add-ins you can try, and even fruits such as blueberries will work. The combination given here will help get you started.

1 tablespoon olive oil
5 turkey sausage patties, crumbled
2 cups frozen hash browns
1 medium onion, cut into ¼-inch dice
6 sweet mini peppers, thinly sliced
4 cups coarsely chopped baby spinach
½ teaspoon sea salt
¼ teaspoon freshly ground black pepper
6 large eggs
2 cups carton egg whites
1¼ cups shredded sharp cheddar cheese

1. Heat the oil in a large cast-iron skillet over medium heat. Add the sausage and cook until browned, about 5 minutes.
2. Add the hash browns, onion, sweet peppers, and spinach and cook, stirring about every 30 seconds, until the hash browns have thawed and the vegetables are soft, about 10 minutes.
3. Add the salt, black pepper, eggs, and egg whites and scramble the eggs into the mixture. Scramble every 30 seconds until the eggs have cooked, about 10 minutes.
4. Remove from the heat and immediately evenly divide into each of 5 single-compartment meal prep containers. Top each container with ¼ cup of cheese. Cover. Store in the refrigerator until needed.

Reheat: From the refrigerator, with the lid cracked, heat in the microwave for 2 minutes. Allow to rest, covered, for 30 seconds before eating.

Per serving: Calories: 405, Total fat: 21g, Total carbs: 22g, Sugar: 4g, Protein: 32g, Fiber: 2g, Sodium: 867mg

Mixed Berry Power Smoothie

GLUTEN-FREE, POST-WORKOUT, STRENGTH, STRENGTH/CARDIO, VEGAN

PREP TIME: 5 MINUTES • **MAKES 2 SERVINGS**

This recipe uses frozen fruit to create a milkshake-like mouthfeel. The addition of plant-based protein makes this smoothie an excellent and refreshing way to recover from a sweaty workout. The berries and spinach give your body a nice antioxidant boost as well.

2 cups frozen mixed berries
2 cups unsweetened almond milk
2 cups baby spinach
2 scoops vanilla plant-based protein powder
8 ice cubes

1. In a blender, combine the berries, milk, spinach, protein powder, and ice cubes and blend on high until smooth, about 1 minute.
2. Drink immediately or freeze any unused portion(s) in a freezer- and microwave-safe prep container.

Reheat: From frozen, heat in the microwave for 2 minutes at 50 percent power. Stir and enjoy. If it still isn't thawed enough to stir, heat on full power an additional 30 seconds.

Substitution Tip: Vanilla whey-based protein powder can be used as well as cow's milk or any milk alternative.

Per serving: Calories: 263, Total fat: 5g, Total carbs: 31g, Sugar: 19g, Protein: 23g, Fiber: 5g, Sodium: 522mg

Peach and Chia Smoothie

CARDIO, GLUTEN-FREE, NUT-FREE, PRE-WORKOUT, VEGAN

PREP TIME: 5 MINUTES • **MAKES:** 2 SERVINGS

This quick and delicious smoothie is a great way to fuel your cardio workouts and a great way to use up frozen overripe bananas. And your blender does all the work!

2 fresh or frozen medium bananas
2 cups sliced frozen peaches
2 cups spinach
2 cups unsweetened plant-based milk
2 tablespoons chia seeds
1 cup water (if using fresh bananas, use 8 ice cubes instead)

1. In a blender, combine the bananas, peaches, spinach, milk, chia seeds, and water and blend on high until smooth, about 1 minute.
2. Drink immediately or freeze any unused portion(s) in a freezer- and microwave-safe prep container.

Reheat: From frozen, heat in the microwave for 2 minutes at 50 percent power. Stir and enjoy. If it still isn't thawed enough to stir, heat on full power an additional 30 seconds.

Per serving: Calories: 268, Total fat: 7g, Total carbs: 52g, Sugar: 29g, Protein: 6g, Fiber: 13g, Sodium: 205mg

Peanut Butter and Banana Smoothie

GLUTEN-FREE, POST-WORKOUT, STRENGTH, STRENGTH/CARDIO, VEGAN

PREP TIME: 5 MINUTES • **MAKES 2 SERVINGS**

If you're a fan of peanut butter milkshakes, this is a nutritious way to experience the same flavor sensation at just a fraction of the calories. This smoothie also includes vegan protein powder to keep you feeling satisfied longer or for use as a post-workout snack. I always have a bag of ripe bananas in my freezer since they're a creamy addition to any smoothie.

2 frozen ripe bananas

2 cups unsweetened almond milk

3 tablespoons creamy peanut butter

2 scoops vanilla plant-based protein powder

8 ice cubes

1. In a blender, combine the bananas, milk, peanut butter, protein powder, and ice cubes and blend on high until smooth, about 1 minute.
2. Drink immediately or freeze any unused portion(s) in a freezer- and microwave-safe prep container.

Reheat: From frozen, heat in the microwave for 2 minutes at 50 percent power. Stir and enjoy. If it still isn't thawed enough to stir, heat on full power an additional 30 seconds.

Substitution Tip: Peanut butter can be swapped for almond butter and any milk alternative can be used.

Per serving: Calories: 434, Total fat: 18g, Total carbs: 46g, Sugar: 25g, Protein: 28g, Fiber: 6g, Sodium: 585mg

Strawberry and Chia Smoothie

CARDIO, GLUTEN-FREE, NUT-FREE, POST-WORKOUT, STRENGTH/CARDIO, VEGETARIAN

PREP TIME: 5 MINUTES • **MAKES 2 SERVINGS**

Chia seeds are a great addition to smoothies because, although tiny, they're very nutritious. They are high in omega-3s, fiber, and essential minerals as well as some protein. They don't provide any flavor so they can be blended into any smoothie for an instant nutrient boost.

2 cups frozen strawberries
1 cup vanilla Greek yogurt
2 cups baby spinach
2 tablespoons chia seeds
1 cup water
8 ice cubes

1. In a blender, combine the strawberries, yogurt, spinach, chia seeds, water, and ice cubes and blend on high until smooth, about 1 minute.
2. Drink immediately or freeze any unused portion(s) in a freezer- and microwave-safe prep container.

Ingredient Tip: Chia thickens liquids as it rests, so thin the smoothie out, 1 tablespoon at a time, with water or milk if desired.

Reheat: From frozen, heat in the microwave for 2 minutes at 50 percent power. Stir and enjoy. If it still isn't thawed enough to stir, heat on full power an additional 30 seconds.

Per serving: Calories: 269, Total fat: 8g, Total carbs: 37g, Sugar: 20g, Protein: 14g, Fiber: 10g, Sodium: 69mg

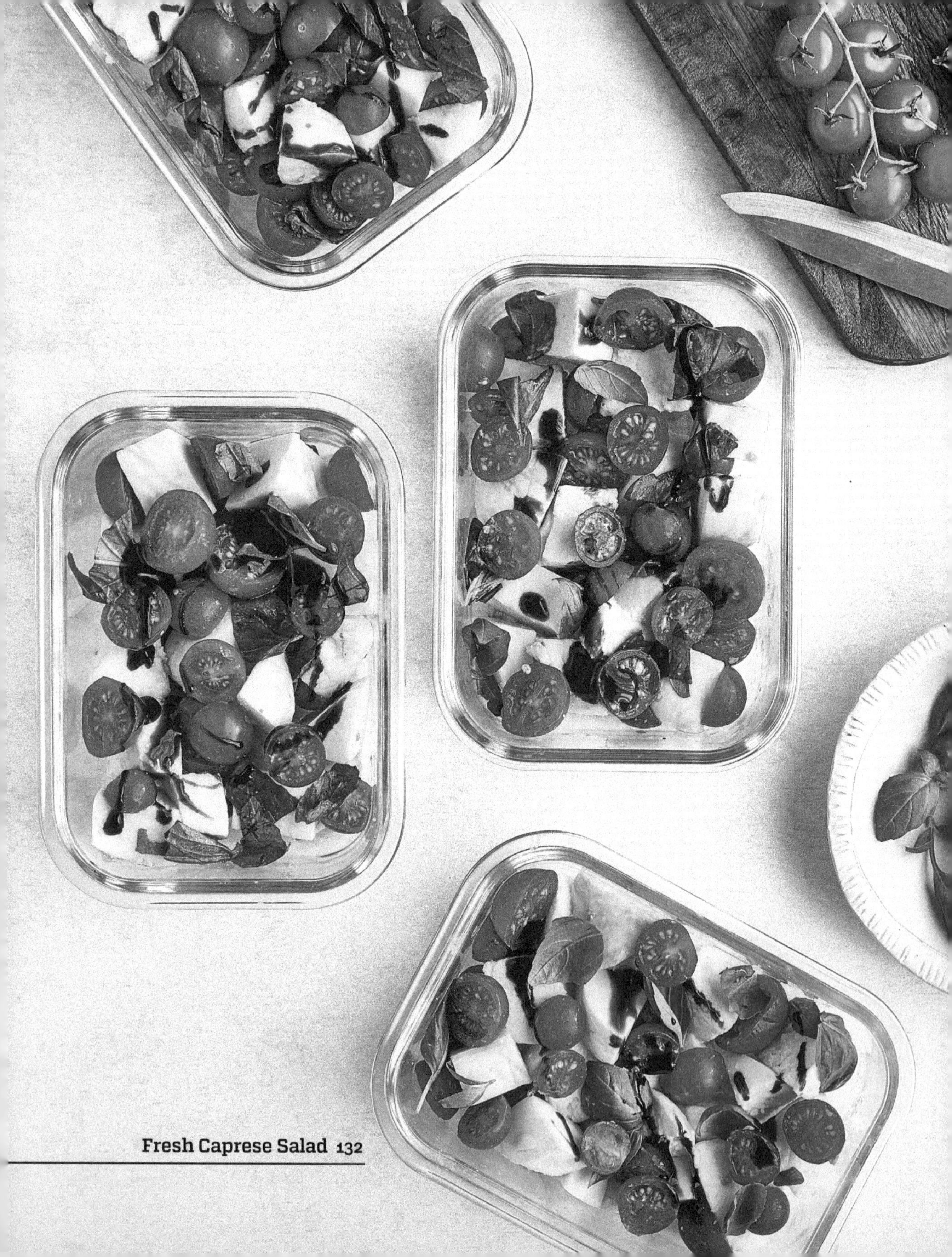

Fresh Caprese Salad 132

CHAPTER SEVEN

POWER SNACKS AND SIDES

Savory Roasted Root Vegetables

CARDIO, GLUTEN-FREE, NUT-FREE, VEGAN

PREP TIME: 15 MINUTES / **COOK TIME:** 50 MINUTES • **MAKES 5 (1-CUP) SERVINGS**

Roasted root vegetables are so versatile. They make a great side dish, a nutritious topping for a big salad, or a healthy addition to a rice bowl. This recipe is featured in both the Quinoa Harvest Bowl with Balsamic Glaze (page 92) and the Roasted Veggie Bowl with Grilled Chicken (page 89).

4 medium (5-inch) sweet potatoes, cut into 1-inch cubes

4 medium (4-inch) yellow potatoes, cut into 1-inch cubes

1 large beet, peeled and cut into 1-inch cubes

1 (16-ounce) bag baby carrots

2 tablespoons olive oil

1 tablespoon garlic powder

1 teaspoon sea salt

¼ teaspoon freshly ground black pepper

¼ cup balsamic vinegar

1. Preheat the oven to 375°F. Line a baking sheet with parchment paper.
2. In a large bowl, combine the sweet potatoes, yellow potatoes, beet, and baby carrots.
3. Add the oil, garlic powder, salt, pepper, and vinegar. Stir to coat the vegetables thoroughly.
4. Spread the vegetables out evenly on the prepared baking sheet and put on the middle rack of the oven. Bake for 25 minutes.
5. Flip the vegetables using a spatula, then return to the oven for about another 25 minutes, or until the vegetables give when pierced.
6. Use in recipes or store until needed in the refrigerator for up to 1 week or in the freezer for a few months.

Reheat: From the refrigerator, with the lid cracked, heat in the microwave for 90 seconds. From frozen, heat for 2 minutes at 50 percent power and then another 45 seconds at full power.

Per serving: Calories: 329, Total fat: 6g, Total carbs: 65g, Sugar: 14g, Protein: 6g, Fiber: 9g, Sodium: 637mg

Roasted Garden Vegetables

CARDIO, GLUTEN-FREE, NUT-FREE, VEGAN

PREP TIME: 10 MINUTES / **COOK TIME:** 30 MINUTES • **MAKES 5 (1-CUP) SERVINGS**

Roasting garden vegetables gives them a whole new flavor profile for a great side dish, a nutritious topping for a big salad, or a hearty addition to a rice bowl. This recipe is featured in both the Quinoa Harvest Bowl with Balsamic Glaze (page 92) and the Roasted Veggie Bowl with Grilled Chicken (page 89). Roasted garden vegetables contain a lot of fiber and plenty of vitamins and antioxidants.

4 cups broccoli florets
4 cups cauliflower florets
10 sweet mini peppers, halved lengthwise
1 large red onion, cut into wedges
2 tablespoons olive oil
1 tablespoon garlic powder
1 teaspoon sea salt
¼ teaspoon freshly ground black pepper
¼ cup balsamic vinegar

1. Preheat the oven to 375°F. Line a baking sheet with parchment paper.
2. In a large bowl, combine the broccoli, cauliflower, sweet peppers, and onion.
3. Add the oil, garlic powder, salt, black pepper, and vinegar and stir to coat the vegetables thoroughly.
4. Spread the vegetables out evenly on the prepared baking sheet and bake for about 30 minutes, or until the florets give when pierced.
5. Use in recipes or store until needed in the refrigerator for up to 1 week or in the freezer for 2 months.

Reheat: From the refrigerator, with the lid cracked, heat in the microwave for 45 seconds. From frozen, heat for 1 minute at 50 percent power and then another 30 seconds at full power.

Per serving: Calories: 130, Total fat: 5g, Total carbs: 16g, Sugar: 8g, Protein: 5g, Fiber: 5g, Sodium: 509mg

Easy Salsa Fresca with Baked Tortilla Chips

CARDIO, GLUTEN-FREE, NUT-FREE, VEGAN

PREP TIME: 15 MINUTES • **MAKES 5 SERVINGS**

Salsa fresca doesn't just have to be something you enjoy at your favorite Mexican restaurant; it can be a healthy snack you can make quickly at home anytime. This flavorful dip is high in nutrition, and eating it with baked tortilla chips makes this snack a lot more calorie- and macro-friendly.

6 medium ripe tomatoes, cut into ¼-inch dice
1 medium onion, cut into ¼-inch dice
1 fresh jalapeño or 1 pickled jalapeño, finely chopped, or more as desired
¼ cup finely chopped fresh cilantro
Juice of 1 lime
2 teaspoons garlic powder
1 teaspoon sea salt
¼ teaspoon freshly ground black pepper
1 (10-ounce) bag baked tortilla chips

1. In a medium bowl, combine the tomatoes, onion, jalapeño, cilantro, lime juice, garlic powder, salt, and pepper. Mix until uniform.
2. If using this to meal prep, evenly divide into single-serve prep containers. Cover. Store in the refrigerator until needed.
3. Prep the chips by placing 1 to 2 servings in a separate prep container or resealable plastic bag.

Ingredient Tip: Using pickled jalapeños can give you more control over the "heat" since they come in different varieties. With fresh ones, the heat can vary.

Per serving: Calories: 281, Total fat: 6g, Total carbs: 52g, Sugar: 6g, Protein: 7g, Fiber: 8g, Sodium: 717mg

Quick-Pickled Garden Vegetables

GLUTEN-FREE, NUT-FREE, VEGAN

PREP TIME: 15 MINUTES, PLUS 48 HOURS TO PICKLE / **COOK TIME:** 10 MINUTES

MAKES 8 SERVINGS

Raw vegetables are nutritious and a great way to increase your micronutrient intake. However, sometimes a person just wants a little more flavor. Instead of dipping them in processed dressing such as ranch, why not pickle them instead? This quick-pickling method doesn't require all the steps traditional pickling requires.

3 pounds garden vegetables, cut into small pieces (e.g., broccoli, cauliflower, sweet mini peppers, cucumber, hot peppers, squash)

4 garlic cloves, crushed

2 teaspoons dried basil

2 teaspoons dried dill

1 teaspoon whole peppercorns

1½ tablespoons sea salt

2 tablespoons sugar

2 cups apple cider vinegar

2 cups water

1. Into 4 jars, stuff the vegetables.
2. Evenly divide the garlic, basil, dill, and peppercorns into each of the jars.
3. In a saucepan over medium heat, bring the salt, sugar, vinegar, and water to a boil, about 10 minutes.
4. Pour the hot liquid over the contents in each jar, stopping a half inch from the top. Seal with the lid and allow to cool at room temperature.
5. Store the jars in the refrigerator and allow to pickle for at least 48 hours before eating.
6. The pickled vegetables will last for up to 2 months in the refrigerator.

Substitution Tip: Many different vegetables can be used with this recipe, so feel free to experiment.

Per serving: Calories: 76, Total fat: 1g, Total carbs: 14g, Sugar: 7g, Protein: 4g, Fiber: 4g, Sodium: 1,361mg

Fresh Caprese Salad

GLUTEN-FREE, NUT-FREE, STRENGTH, STRENGTH/CARDIO, VEGETARIAN

PREP TIME: 15 MINUTES • **MAKES 5 SERVINGS**

Caprese salad has a great blend of flavors and provides a terrific snack, appetizer, or side dish. You can eat it by itself or on top of some whole-grain toast. This is a tasty way to recharge after your workout session. To make your own balsamic glaze, see the tip in the Quinoa Harvest Bowl with Balsamic Glaze recipe (page 92).

16 ounces fresh 2% (low-fat) mozzarella cheese, cut into 1-inch cubes

½ cup coarsely chopped fresh basil

16 ounces cherry tomatoes, halved

½ teaspoon sea salt

5 tablespoons prepared balsamic glaze

1. In a medium bowl, combine the mozzarella, basil, tomatoes, and salt. Gently stir.
2. Evenly divide the salad into each of 5 single-compartment prep containers and drizzle the balsamic evenly over each.
3. Cover. Store in the refrigerator until needed.

Ingredient Tip: Using cherry or grape tomatoes instead of regular tomatoes gives the caprese salad a sweeter taste. Make sure the tomatoes are ripe. If they don't taste sweet, let them sit on your kitchen counter for a few days.

Per serving: Calories: 311, Total fat: 20g, Total carbs: 12g, Sugar: 11g, Protein: 17g, Fiber: 1g, Sodium: 518mg

Oven-Baked Beans

DAIRY-FREE, GLUTEN-FREE, NUT-FREE, STRENGTH/CARDIO, VEGETARIAN

PREP TIME: 10 MINUTES / **COOK TIME:** 40 MINUTES • **MAKES 5 SERVINGS**

It can be tempting to just grab a can of baked beans off the grocery store shelf, but taking a few minutes to make your own isn't only healthier, it's also much tastier. Here's an easy baked bean recipe that you can use as a side dish or snack.

1 (15-ounce) can white beans, drained
1 (15-ounce) can black beans, drained
1 (15-ounce) can red beans, drained
1 medium onion, cut into ¼-inch dice
1 green bell pepper, cut into ¼-inch dice
1 (15-ounce) can tomato sauce
5 tablespoons brown sugar
1 tablespoon yellow mustard
1 tablespoon gluten-free Worcestershire sauce
1 teaspoon sea salt
1 teaspoon garlic powder
¼ teaspoon freshly ground black pepper

1. Preheat the oven to 350°F.
2. In a large bowl, combine the beans, onion, bell pepper, tomato sauce, sugar, mustard, Worcestshire sauce, salt, garlic powder, and black pepper and mix until uniform.
3. Transfer the beans to a baking dish and bake, uncovered, for about 40 minutes, or until the beans are warmed through.
4. Let cool for 10 minutes.
5. If using this recipe for prepping, divide equally into each of 5 single-compartment prep containers. Cover. Store in the refrigerator until needed.

Reheat: From the refrigerator, with the lid cracked, heat in the microwave for 2 minutes, stirring between each 1-minute increment.

Per serving: Calories: 317, Total fat: 2g, Total carbs: 62g, Sugar: 15g, Protein: 16g, Fiber: 19g, Sodium: 958mg

Marinated Carrots

CARDIO, DAIRY-FREE, GLUTEN-FREE, NUT-FREE, VEGETARIAN

PREP TIME: 15 MINUTES, PLUS OVERNIGHT TO MARINATE / **COOK TIME:** 20 MINUTES

MAKES 6 SERVINGS

Carrots are great as a side dish, and it's always good to have a few different ways to enjoy them. This marinated version gives them a great tangy flavor and makes a perfect side dish or even a quick pre-workout snack.

2 pounds fresh carrots, washed and thinly sliced

1 (10-ounce) can condensed tomato soup

½ cup honey

¼ cup olive oil

¾ cup apple cider vinegar

¼ teaspoon freshly ground black pepper

1 medium onion, cut into ¼-inch dice

1 green bell pepper, cut into ¼-inch dice

1. In a medium pot over medium-high heat, cover the carrots with water and bring to a boil. Boil, uncovered, for about 20 minutes, or until the carrots soften.
2. While the carrots are cooking, in a microwave-safe bowl, stir together the tomato soup, honey, oil, vinegar, and black pepper.
3. Heat in the microwave for 1 minute, stir, then heat for another minute. Repeat until the mixture is hot and steaming. Set aside.
4. When the carrots are cooked, add them to the sauce along with the onion and bell pepper.
5. Evenly divide into each of 6 single-compartment prep containers. Cover. Store in the refrigerator and let marinate overnight. (The sauce is to be eaten with the carrots).

Per serving: Calories: 202, Total fat: 1g, Total carbs: 49g, Sugar: 36g, Protein: 3g, Fiber: 6g, Sodium: 399mg

Nut Butter and Assorted Fruits

GLUTEN-FREE, PRE-WORKOUT, STRENGTH/CARDIO, VEGAN

PREP TIME: 5 MINUTES • MAKES 1 SERVING

Here's a super quick snack you can eat before your workout. It contains a great blend of healthy carbs, healthy fats, and some protein. It also has that wonderful salty/sweet flavor that most people crave.

Fruit choices

1 large apple, cut into 4 large wedges
1 large banana, cut into 6 pieces
6 medium strawberries
6 (2-inch) cubes melon

Nut butter choices

2 tablespoons natural salted peanut butter
2 tablespoons natural salted almond butter
2 tablespoons natural cashew butter

Spread an equal amount of nut butter on each piece of fruit. Eat right away or store until needed. (See tip.)

Prep Tip: This can be prepped ahead of time and stored in the refrigerator until needed. Squeeze a little lemon juice over your apples to prevent them from turning brown.

Per serving: Calories: 309, Total fat: 17g, Total carbs: 38g, Sugar: 27g, Protein: 8g, Fiber: 7g, Sodium: 8mg

Quick and Creamy Deviled Eggs

GLUTEN-FREE, NUT-FREE, POST-WORKOUT, STRENGTH, VEGETARIAN

PREP TIME: 20 MINUTES / **COOK TIME:** 15 MINUTES • **MAKES 24 DEVILED EGGS**

Why settle for boring hard-boiled eggs when, in just a few more steps, you can experience flavorful creamy deviled eggs instead? I've tweaked it to make it a little healthier, using light mayonnaise.

12 large eggs
1 cup light mayonnaise
1 tablespoon yellow mustard
½ teaspoon sea salt
Paprika, for garnish

1. In a 2-quart pot over high heat, cover the eggs with water and bring to a boil. Reduce the heat to medium and boil, uncovered, for 12 minutes.
2. Remove from the heat, drain off the hot water, and fill the pot with cold water. Allow the eggs to rest in the cold water for 10 minutes.
3. While the eggs are resting, in a small bowl, combine the mayonnaise, mustard, and salt and mix together until creamy.
4. Peel the eggs. Slice each egg in half and use a small spoon to remove the yolks. Place the yolks in the bowl with the mayonnaise mixture.
5. Arrange the empty egg white halves on a plate.
6. Use a fork or potato masher to mash the yolks into the mayonnaise mixture, then stir vigorously until creamy.
7. Evenly divide the egg yolk mixture into each of the 24 egg white halves. Sprinkle with paprika.
8. Place 4 deviled egg halves in each of 6 prep containers. Cover. Store in the refrigerator until needed. Freezing is not recommended.

Prep Tip: If you have a hand mixer, use this to mix the egg yolks and mayonnaise mixture together. It makes it both easier and creamier.

Per serving (4 deviled eggs): Calories: 276, Total fat: 21g, Total carbs: 7g, Sugar: 3g, Protein: 13g, Fiber: 0g, Sodium: 600mg

Chicken Salad with Whole-Grain Crackers

NUT-FREE, POST-WORKOUT, STRENGTH, STRENGTH/CARDIO

PREP TIME: 10 MINUTES / **COOK TIME:** 30 MINUTES • **MAKES 5 SERVINGS**

A healthy chicken salad is a satisfying alternative to a protein shake after your workout. Chicken is a higher-quality protein than whey and is more filling than consuming a liquid. I keep this chicken salad recipe on the healthier side by using light mayonnaise and some Greek yogurt for creaminess.

20 ounces boneless, skinless chicken breasts

4 celery stalks, thinly sliced

½ medium red onion, cut into ¼-inch dice

¾ cup light mayonnaise

½ cup low-fat plain Greek yogurt

½ teaspoon sea salt

½ teaspoon paprika

¼ teaspoon freshly ground black pepper

30 whole-grain crackers

1. In a 2-quart pot over high heat, cover the chicken breasts with water and bring to a boil. Reduce the heat to medium and boil, uncovered, for about 25 minutes, or until the chicken breasts are cooked (poached).
2. Remove from the heat, drain, and let cool for 15 minutes.
3. In a medium bowl, shred the chicken using your fingers or 2 forks.
4. Add the celery, onion, mayonnaise, yogurt, salt, paprika, and pepper, and mix until well combined and creamy.
5. Evenly divide the chicken salad into each of 5 single-compartment prep containers. Cover. Store in the refrigerator until needed. Put 6 crackers into each of 5 separate containers or resealable plastic bags.

Substitution Tip: This chicken salad makes a great sandwich. Switch out the crackers for 2 slices of whole-grain bread.

Per serving: Calories: 383, Total fat: 17g, Total carbs: 27g, Sugar: 4g, Protein: 31g, Fiber: 4g, Sodium: 770mg

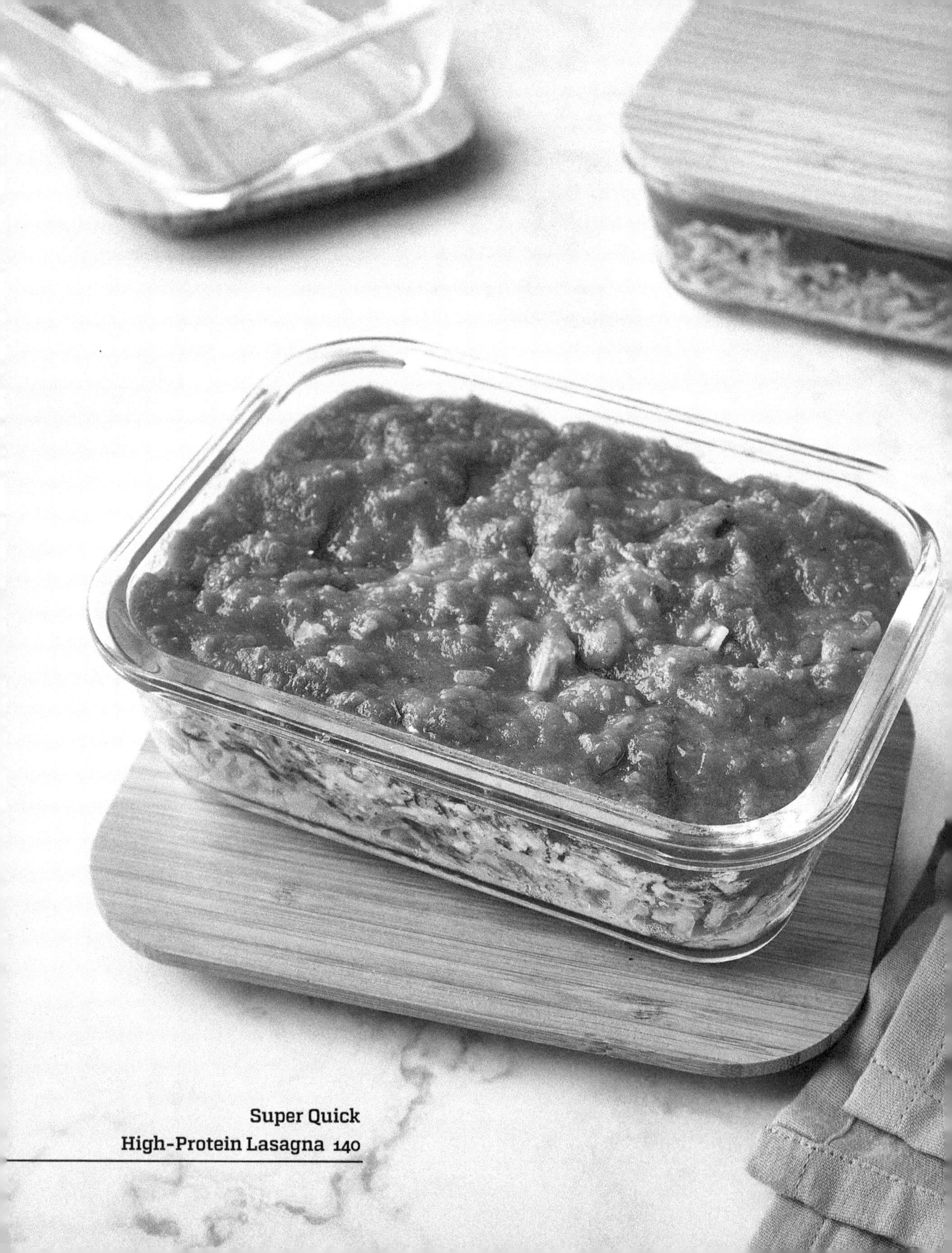

Super Quick
High-Protein Lasagna 140

CHAPTER EIGHT

MIGHTY MAINS

Super Quick High-Protein Lasagna

GLUTEN-FREE, NUT-FREE, POST-WORKOUT, STRENGTH, STRENGTH/CARDIO, VEGETARIAN

PREP TIME: 15 MINUTES / **COOK TIME:** 50 MINUTES • **MAKES 6 SERVINGS**

Lasagna is always a hit, but traditional lasagna is high in calories and takes a while to make. This recipe changes all that. Not only is it healthier, it can also be thrown together quickly. I use chickpea-based pasta to increase the protein content as well as lower-fat cheeses to keep the fat macro in check. There are also some vegetables thrown in to increase the micronutrient profile.

4 quarts water
8 ounces spiral chickpea pasta
2 carrots, shredded
4 cups chopped spinach
16 ounces low-fat cottage cheese
1½ cups low-fat mozzarella cheese, divided
1 tablespoon garlic powder
2 teaspoons Italian seasoning
1 (15-ounce) jar marinara sauce
¼ teaspoon freshly ground black pepper

1. Preheat the oven to 350°F.
2. In a 5-quart pot over high heat, bring the water to a boil. Add the pasta and cook for 5 minutes.
3. Drain the pasta and transfer to a 9-by-13-inch baking pan or casserole dish.
4. In a medium bowl, combine the carrots, spinach, cottage cheese, 1 cup of mozzarella, the garlic powder, and Italian seasoning and stir until uniform.
5. Evenly distribute the cheese mixture over the pasta. Pour the marinara sauce over the cheese and pasta evenly. Sprinkle the remaining ½ cup of mozzarella over the top.
6. Bake for about 45 minutes, or until the cheese is bubbly and browned.

7. Remove from the oven and let cool for 10 minutes.

8. Evenly divide the lasagna into each of 6 single-compartment prep containers. Cover. Store in the refrigerator until needed.

Reheat: From the refrigerator, with the lid cracked, heat in the microwave for 2½ minutes. Let rest 1 minute before eating.

Substitution Tip: You can use traditional low-fat ricotta cheese instead of cottage cheese.

Per serving: Calories: 334, Total fat: 11g, Total carbs: 38g, Sugar: 11g, Protein: 26g, Fiber: 6g, Sodium: 737mg

Tuna Burgers

DAIRY-FREE, NUT-FREE, POST-WORKOUT, STRENGTH

PREP TIME: 10 MINUTES / **COOK TIME:** 30 MINUTES • **MAKES 4 SERVINGS**

High-quality canned tuna is an excellent protein source that also contains omega-3 fatty acids. Here's an easy way to enjoy the benefits. These tuna burgers can be eaten on a whole-grain bun or on top of a big leafy green salad for a lower-carb option.

2 (12-ounce) cans solid white albacore tuna, drained

2 large eggs

2 tablespoons light mayonnaise

½ cup Italian-style bread crumbs

½ teaspoon paprika

¼ teaspoon freshly ground black pepper

Olive oil cooking spray

1. In a medium bowl, combine the tuna, eggs, mayonnaise, bread crumbs, paprika, and pepper. Stir until well combined.
2. Heat a large nonstick skillet over medium heat. Spray the skillet with cooking spray. Using a spoon, make 4 equal-size patties with half the tuna mixture.
3. Cook for about 7 minutes, then flip with a spatula and cook for about 7 more minutes, or until both sides are golden brown. Repeat with the remaining tuna mixture.
4. Place 2 tuna burgers in each of 2 single-compartment prep containers. Cover. Store in the refrigerator until needed.

Reheat: From the refrigerator, with the lid cracked, heat in the microwave for 90 seconds.

Per serving: Calories: 282, Total fat: 9g, Total carbs: 11g, Sugar: 2g, Protein: 36g, Fiber: 1g, Sodium: 770mg

Southwest Green Chile Stew

DAIRY-FREE, GLUTEN-FREE, NUT-FREE, POST-WORKOUT, STRENGTH

PREP TIME: 10 MINUTES / **COOK TIME:** 1 HOUR • **MAKES 6 SERVINGS**

If you've ever been to New Mexico, you'd have seen green chiles on the menu everywhere. Green chiles add a little heat but a lot of flavor. This flavorful stew uses lean pork and potatoes to refuel after working out.

2 pounds lean pork (pork loin or tenderloin), cut into 1- to 2-inch cubes

1 cup water

3 cups chicken broth

1 (15-ounce) can diced tomatoes

2 (7-ounce) cans diced green chiles

1 tablespoon ground cumin

1 tablespoon dried oregano

2 teaspoons garlic powder

2 teaspoons sea salt

½ teaspoon freshly ground black pepper

2 pounds yellow potatoes, cut into 1- to 2-inch cubes

1 (15-ounce) can white beans

4 cups coarsely chopped baby spinach

1 (10-ounce) bag baked tortilla chips, for serving

1. In a 5-quart pot over medium-high heat, brown the pork for about 5 minutes.
2. Reduce the heat to medium and add the water, broth, tomatoes, chiles, cumin, oregano, garlic powder, salt, and black pepper. Bring to a boil, stirring occasionally.
3. When the mixture starts to boil, add the potatoes, beans, and spinach. Bring back to a boil, then reduce the heat to low, cover, and cook for about 45 minutes, or until the pork is cooked.
4. Let cool for 10 minutes. Evenly divide the stew into each of 6 single-compartment prep containers. Cover. Store in the refrigerator or freezer until needed.
5. Evenly divide the tortilla chips into 6 containers or resealable plastic bags.

Reheat: From the refrigerator, with the lid cracked, heat in the microwave for 3 minutes, stirring after each 1-minute increment. From frozen, heat for 2 minutes in the microwave at 50 percent power and then follow the refrigerator directions. Before serving, crumble 1 serving of tortilla chips on top of the stew.

Per serving: Calories: 627, Total fat: 9g, Total carbs: 92g, Sugar: 7g, Protein: 49g, Fiber: 14g, Sodium: 1,848mg

Six-Layer Bake

DAIRY-FREE, GLUTEN-FREE, NUT-FREE, STRENGTH/CARDIO

PREP TIME: 15 MINUTES / **COOK TIME:** 1 HOUR 10 MINUTES • **MAKES 6 SERVINGS**

This is a one-pan casserole-type recipe that's super simple but really delicious. The lean turkey supplies the protein, and your whole foods–based carb source comes from the potatoes and other vegetables. This is a comfort-food recipe that you can eat without guilt as you fuel your body or recover from a fitness session.

2 pounds yellow potatoes, thinly sliced
4 celery stalks, thinly sliced
1 pound 93% lean ground turkey
1 medium sweet onion, thinly sliced
2 green bell peppers, cut into ¼-inch dice
1 (15-ounce) jar marinara sauce

1. Preheat the oven to 350°F. Line a 9-by-13-inch baking pan with parchment paper.
2. Layer the potatoes on the bottom of the pan. Layer in the celery, then the turkey, then the onion, then the bell peppers. Pour the marinara sauce evenly over the top.
3. Bake for 1 hour 10 minutes.
4. Let cool for 10 minutes. Evenly divide into each of 6 single-compartment prep containers. Cover. Store in the refrigerator or freezer until needed.

Reheat: From the refrigerator, with the lid cracked, heat in the microwave for 2 minutes. Let rest 1 minute before eating. From frozen, with the lid cracked, heat for 2 minutes on 50 percent power and then for 2 additional minutes on full power. Allow to rest 1 minute before eating.

Per serving: Calories: 313, Total fat: 8g, Total carbs: 46g, Sugar: 9g, Protein: 19g, Fiber: 4g, Sodium: 337mg

High-Protein Spaghetti and Meatballs

NUT-FREE, POST-WORKOUT, STRENGTH, STRENGTH/CARDIO

PREP TIME: 15 MINUTES / **COOK TIME:** 30 MINUTES • **MAKES 4 SERVINGS**

Spaghetti and meatballs is a classic dish that many people have eaten from childhood. My version uses lean turkey for the meatballs and chickpea pasta to create a better balance of macronutrients.

1 pound 93% lean ground turkey
½ cup Italian-style bread crumbs
2 teaspoons garlic powder
½ teaspoon sea salt
¼ teaspoon freshly ground black pepper
2 teaspoons Italian seasoning
2 large eggs
12 ounces chickpea spaghetti
1 (15-ounce) jar marinara sauce
½ cup shredded Parmesan cheese

1. Preheat the oven to 375°F. Line a baking sheet with parchment paper.
2. In a medium bowl, combine the turkey, bread crumbs, garlic powder, salt, pepper, Italian seasoning, and eggs. Mix until smooth.
3. Form the mixture into 16 (1- to 2-inch) balls and spread them evenly on the prepared baking sheet. Bake for about 30 minutes, or until the meatballs brown.
4. While the meatballs are baking, fill a 5-quart pot three-fourths full of water and bring to a boil over high heat.
5. Add the pasta, return to a boil, and cook according to package instructions, about 8 minutes over medium heat, stirring occasionally, or until al dente.
6. Drain the pasta in a colander and rinse with hot tap water.
7. When the meatballs are cooked, evenly divide the pasta into each of 4 single-compartment prep containers. Pour one-fourth of the marinara sauce over each, place 4 meatballs on top, and sprinkle with 2 tablespoons of Parmesan. Store in the refrigerator until needed.

Reheat: From the refrigerator, with the lid cracked, heat for 2½ minutes. Let rest an additional minute before eating.

Per serving: Calories: 662, Total fat: 23g, Total carbs: 71g, Sugar: 13g, Protein: 52g, Fiber: 11g, Sodium: 1,227mg

Savory Lentil Veggie Burgers

CARDIO, NUT-FREE, VEGAN

PREP TIME: 15 MINUTES / **COOK TIME:** 30 MINUTES • **MAKES 4 SERVINGS**

Many plant-based burgers try to imitate the taste of meat, but plant-based burgers can be delicious without the use of meat flavors. This hearty veggie burger recipe is packed with healthy carbs and plant protein to keep your workouts going. Serve on a whole-grain bun, in wraps, or simply by themselves.

2 (15-ounce) cans green lentils, drained
1 cup Italian-style bread crumbs
1 cup vegetable stock
2 tablespoons ground flaxseed
2 carrots, shredded
3 cups coarsely chopped baby spinach
1 small beet, shredded
1 teaspoon garlic powder
1 teaspoon sea salt
¼ teaspoon freshly ground black pepper
Olive oil cooking spray

1. In a medium bowl, combine the lentils, bread crumbs, stock, flaxseed, carrots, spinach, beet, garlic powder, salt, and pepper. Stir well to make all the mixture uniform and to activate the flaxseed.
2. Spray a large nonstick skillet with cooking spray and heat over medium heat.
3. Use a spoon to dollop batter into the skillet to form 3- to 4-inch-diameter patties.
4. Cook the patties for 5 to 6 minutes, then flip each burger and cook for an additional 5 to 6 minutes. Repeat for any remaining batter, for a total of 8 burgers.
5. Place 2 burgers in each of 4 single-compartment prep containers. Store in the refrigerator until needed. They can also be wrapped individually in plastic wrap and frozen.

Reheat: From the refrigerator, with the lid cracked, heat in the microwave for 1½ minutes. From frozen, remove the plastic wrap and heat, wrapped in a damp paper towel, at 50 percent power for 1 minute then for 1 minute at full power.

Per serving: Calories: 374, Total fat: 3g, Total carbs: 64g, Sugar: 7g, Protein: 22g, Fiber: 16g, Sodium: 1,213mg

Roasted Pork Tenderloin and Gold Potatoes

DAIRY-FREE, GLUTEN-FREE, NUT-FREE, POST-WORKOUT, STRENGTH, STRENGTH/CARDIO

PREP TIME: 10 MINUTES / **COOK TIME:** 40 MINUTES • **MAKES 4 SERVINGS**

When considering protein options, pork is often overlooked, because many cuts tend to be fatty. However, pork tenderloin is an exception—it's a lean cut that is also very tender. Here's an easy recipe for a healthy protein-rich post-workout meal. Serve with a leafy green salad.

1 tablespoon garlic powder
1 teaspoon paprika
2 teaspoons sea salt
¼ teaspoon freshly ground black pepper
1½ pounds pork tenderloin
2 tablespoons olive oil, divided
2 pounds yellow potatoes, cut into 1- to 2-inch cubes

1. Preheat the oven to 400°F. Line a 9-by-13-inch baking pan with parchment paper.
2. In a small bowl, combine the garlic powder, paprika, salt, and pepper.
3. Coat the tenderloin with 1 tablespoon of oil and then half of the seasoning mix.
4. Place the tenderloin in the center of the prepared pan.
5. In a medium bowl, combine the potatoes and remaining 1 tablespoon of oil. Stir the potatoes to coat. Add the remaining seasoning mix and stir to coat the potatoes evenly.
6. Arrange the potatoes around the tenderloin. Bake for about 40 minutes, until cooked through or a thermometer reads 145°F.
7. Remove from the oven and let rest for 10 minutes.
8. Evenly divide the pork and potatoes into each of 4 single-compartment prep containers. Cover. Store in the refrigerator until needed.

Reheat: From the refrigerator, with the lid cracked, heat in the microwave for 2 minutes. Allow to rest 1 minute before digging in.

Per serving: Calories: 461, Total fat: 11g, Total carbs: 54g, Sugar: 2g, Protein: 40g, Fiber: 3g, Sodium: 1,272mg

Oven Chicken and Dumplings

NUT-FREE, POST-WORKOUT, STRENGTH, STRENGTH/CARDIO

PREP TIME: 15 MINUTES / **COOK TIME:** 45 MINUTES • **MAKES 4 SERVINGS**

Chicken and dumplings is wonderful comfort food. This recipe is my healthier take on the classic recipe many of us have enjoyed eating. It's made in the oven for simplicity and is great for meal prep because it stores well in the refrigerator.

24 ounces boneless, skinless chicken breast, cut into 1- to 2-inch cubes
3 cups chicken broth
1 medium onion, chopped
1 (16-ounce) bag frozen mixed peas and carrots
2 cups whole wheat flour
2 teaspoons baking powder
1 teaspoon sea salt
¼ cup olive oil
¾ cup milk or plant-based alternative

1. Preheat the oven to 350°F.
2. In a 9-by-13-inch baking pan, spread the chicken in an even layer. Add the broth, onion, and peas/carrots, and stir to evenly disperse.
3. In a medium bowl, combine the flour, baking powder, salt, oil, and milk. Stir until a wet dough forms, about 1 minute.
4. Use a small spoon to drop dollops of batter evenly on top of the chicken and vegetables. Do not stir the batter in.
5. Bake for about 45 minutes, or until the dumplings are cooked and browned.
6. Remove from the oven and let cool for 15 minutes.
7. Evenly divide into each of 4 single-compartment prep containers. Cover. Store in the refrigerator until needed.

Reheat: From the refrigerator, with the lid cracked, heat in the microwave for 2 minutes. Let rest 1 minute before eating.

Per serving: Calories: 621, Total fat: 21g, Total carbs: 61g, Sugar: 5g, Protein: 52g, Fiber: 10g, Sodium: 1,709mg

Jambalaya-Inspired Rice

DAIRY-FREE, GLUTEN-FREE, NUT-FREE, POST-WORKOUT, STRENGTH/CARDIO

PREP TIME: 15 MINUTES / **COOK TIME:** 45 MINUTES • **MAKES 6 SERVINGS**

This Creole-inspired rice is modified to be a little more macro-friendly than traditional jambalaya and has been simplified to make it easier for you to prepare, but without sacrificing all the delicious flavors this dish offers. You can control the heat and make it as spicy or mild as you want.

1 tablespoon olive oil
12 ounces (smoke-flavored) gluten-free chicken sausage, sliced
1 pound boneless, skinless chicken breast, cut into 1- to 2-inch cubes
2 tablespoons Cajun seasoning
1 medium onion, cut into ¼-inch dice
1 green bell pepper, cut into ¼-inch dice
1 red bell pepper, cut into ¼-inch dice
3 celery stalks, thinly sliced
1 (15-ounce) can crushed tomatoes
1 tablespoon garlic powder
½ teaspoon freshly ground black pepper
1 teaspoon hot sauce
1 teaspoon dried oregano
1 teaspoon dried thyme
3 teaspoons Worcestershire sauce
3 cups chicken broth
1½ cups brown rice, rinsed well
1 pound frozen peeled, deveined, tail-off raw shrimp

1. In a 5-quart pot, heat the oil over medium heat. Add the sausage, chicken breast, and Cajun seasoning and sauté for about 5 minutes, or until the meat begins to brown.
2. Add the onion, bell peppers, and celery and sauté for about another 5 minutes, or until the vegetables start to soften.
3. Add the tomatoes, garlic powder, black pepper, hot sauce, oregano, thyme, Worcestershire sauce, broth, and rice and stir.
4. Increase the heat and bring the mixture to a boil. Let boil for 5 minutes.
5. Cover, reduce the heat to low, and simmer for about 25 minutes, or until the liquid is almost completely absorbed.
6. Add the shrimp, cover, and cook for about another 5 minutes, or until the shrimp is transluscent and the liquid is completely absorbed.

>>

7. Remove from the heat and let rest for 15 minutes.
8. Evenly divide the jambalaya into each of 6 single-compartment prep containers. Store in the refrigerator or freezer until needed.

Reheat: From the refrigerator, with the lid cracked, heat in the microwave for 2½ minutes. From frozen, with the lid cracked, heat for 2 minutes at 50 percent power and then another 2 minutes at full power. For both methods, let rest 1 minute before eating.

Per serving: Calories: 507, Total fat: 14g, Total carbs: 53g, Sugar: 7g, Protein: 44g, Fiber: 5g, Sodium: 1,593mg

High-Protein Pasta with Meat Sauce

GLUTEN-FREE, NUT-FREE, STRENGTH, STRENGTH/CARDIO

PREP TIME: 15 MINUTES / **COOK TIME:** 20 MINUTES • **MAKES 4 SERVINGS**

This is another classic dish that I've modified to be high in protein and lower in carbs. Chickpea pasta increases the protein content, and lean turkey sausage improves the flavor profile. If you can, serve this with a fresh side salad.

1 pound 93% lean grass-fed ground beef
4 ounces turkey sausage
1 teaspoon garlic powder
1 (15-ounce) jar marinara sauce
4 cups coarsely chopped baby spinach
12 ounces chickpea or lentil pasta (spaghetti or linguini)
4 tablespoons grated Parmesan cheese, for garnish

1. Fill a 5-quart pot three-fourths full of water and bring to a boil on high heat.
2. While the water is heating, in a 2 quart-pot on medium heat, brown the beef and turkey, stirring regularly and breaking up the chunks of meat, about 10 minutes.
3. Add the garlic powder, marinara, and spinach to the meat. Stir until combined. Reduce the heat to low and cover.
4. Add the pasta to the boiling water in the 5-quart pot and cook for 9 minutes.
5. Drain the pasta and rinse with hot tap water.
6. Evenly divide the pasta into each of 4 single-compartment prep containers and top each with one-fourth of the meat sauce.
7. Top each with 1 tablespoon of Parmesan. Store in the refrigerator until needed.

Reheat: From the refrigerator, with the lid cracked, heat in the microwave for 2½ minutes. Let rest 1 minute before eating.

Per serving: Calories: 615, Total fat: 20g, Total carbs: 63g, Sugar: 11g, Protein: 54g, Fiber: 10g, Sodium: 851mg

Grilled Chicken Skewers with Lemon Garlic Quinoa

DAIRY-FREE, GLUTEN-FREE, NUT-FREE, STRENGTH, STRENGTH/CARDIO

PREP TIME: 15 MINUTES, PLUS 30 MINUTES TO MARINATE / **COOK TIME:** 40 MINUTES

MAKES 4 SERVINGS

This is a perfect dish to enjoy on a hot day, or anytime really, because of the great combination of lean protein, fresh vegetables, and healthy carbs. It's best cooked on a gas grill, but they can be cooked in a pan or on a griddle as well. Make sure to soak 16 skewers in water for 30 minutes before use so they don't burn.

1 cup Italian dressing
1½ pounds boneless, skinless chicken breast, cut into 2-inch cubes
2 cups water
1 cup quinoa, rinsed well
Juice of 1 lemon
1 tablespoon garlic powder
1 teaspoon sea salt
16 sweet mini peppers
16 whole white button mushrooms
2 medium zucchini, cut into 16 slices
1 medium red onion, cut into 16 wedges
1 tablespoon olive oil
1 teaspoon seasoned salt

1. In a small bowl, combine the dressing and chicken. Cover and marinate in the refrigerator for at least 30 minutes.
2. In a 2-quart pot over high heat, combine the water, quinoa, lemon juice, garlic powder, and sea salt. Bring to a boil, then cover, reduce the heat to low, and simmer for about 25 minutes, until the liquid is absorbed.
3. In a medium bowl, add the peppers, mushrooms, zucchini, and onion. Add the oil and seasoned salt and stir until the vegetables are evenly coated.
4. When the quinoa is done, leave covered and set aside.
5. Preheat the gas grill to medium heat.
6. Assemble the skewers by alternating pieces of chicken and vegetables.
7. Cook on the grill, rotating to cook each side for about 3 minutes, for a total of 12 minutes, until the chicken is cooked and browned. If using a nonstick pan or griddle, cook over medium heat using the same time frame.

8. Evenly divide the quinoa into each of 4 single-compartment prep containers. To each container, add the chicken and vegetables from 4 skewers on top of the quinoa. Store in the refrigerator until needed.

Reheat: From the refrigerator, with the lid cracked, heat in the microwave for 2 minutes. Let rest 1 minute before serving.

Per serving: Calories: 523, Total fat: 12g, Total carbs: 55g, Sugar: 20g, Protein: 48g, Fiber: 8g, Sodium: 1,801mg

Creamy Black Bean Soup

CARDIO, GLUTEN-FREE, NUT-FREE, VEGAN

PREP TIME: 10 MINUTES / **COOK TIME:** 25 MINUTES • **MAKES 6 SERVINGS**

This black bean soup is made deliciously creamy by using a blender to process all the ingredients. The result is a thick, flavorful soup that's rich in plant-based protein and healthy carbs—perfect for your fitness goals.

3 cups vegetable broth
1 medium sweet onion, coarsely chopped
½ cup prepared roasted red peppers
2 (15-ounce) cans black beans
2 cups baby spinach
1 tablespoon garlic powder
¼ teaspoon freshly ground black pepper
1 teaspoon ground cumin
¼ cup balsamic vinegar

1. In a blender, combine the broth, onion, red peppers, black beans, spinach, garlic powder, black pepper, cumin, and vinegar and blend on high for 2 minutes until smooth and creamy.
2. Transfer to a 5-quart pot over medium heat and heat until hot and steaming, stirring occasionally, about 25 minutes.
3. Evenly divide the soup into each of 6 single-compartment prep containers. Cover. Store in the refrigerator until needed.

Reheat: From the refrigerator, with the lid cracked, heat in the microwave for 3 minutes, stirring after each 1-minute increment.

Per serving: Calories: 165, Total fat: 1g, Total carbs: 33g, Sugar: 5g, Protein: 10g, Fiber: 12g, Sodium: 826mg

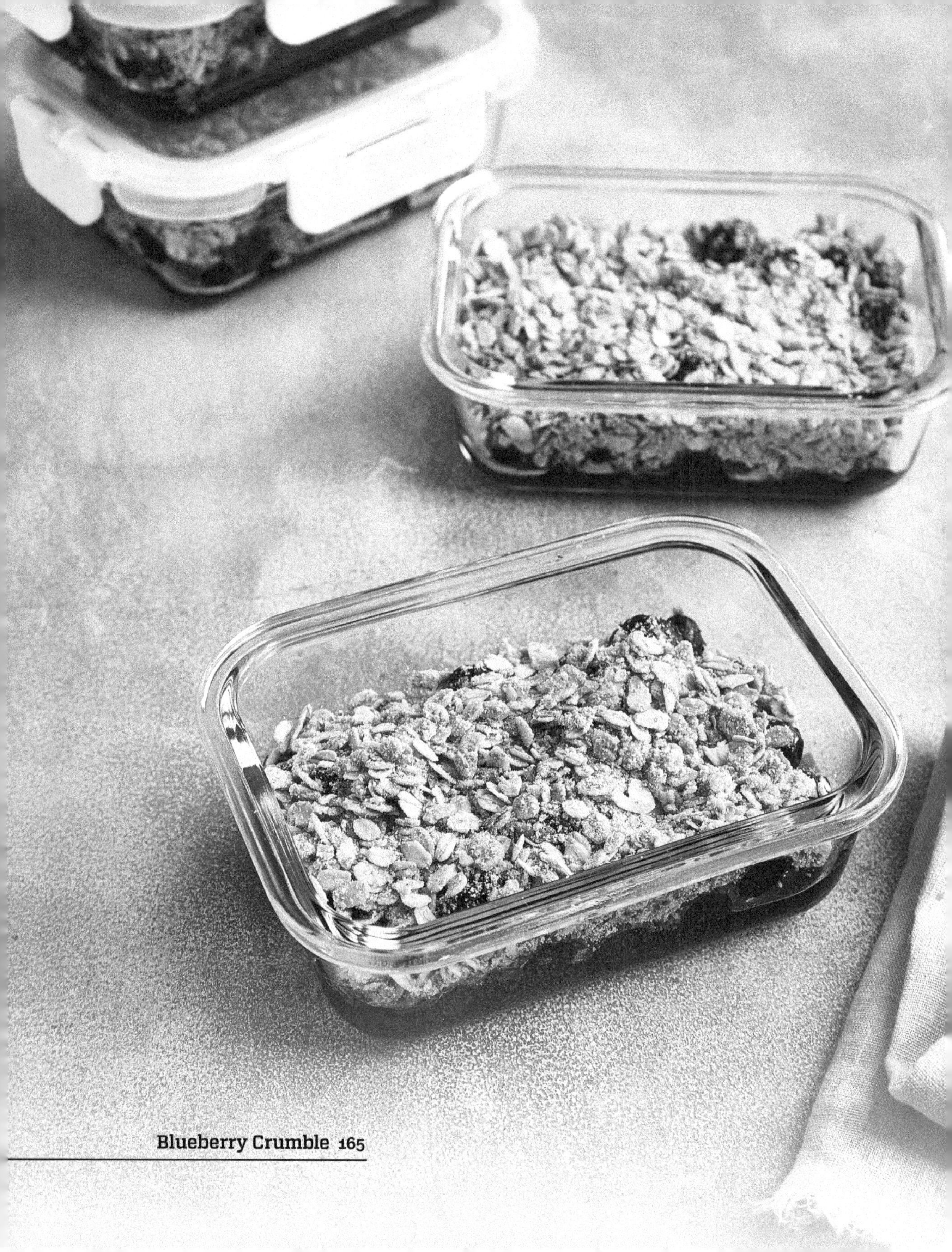

Blueberry Crumble

CHAPTER NINE

SOMETHING SWEET

Peanut Butter Honey Protein Balls

DAIRY-FREE, GLUTEN-FREE, POST-WORKOUT, STRENGTH, STRENGTH/CARDIO, VEGETARIAN

PREP TIME: 10 MINUTES • **MAKES 20 BALLS**

This quick dessert recipe provides not only a great post-workout treat but also a high-protein snack anytime you need a fast and convenient energy boost. The balls have a nice blend of protein, carbs, and fat to keep you feeling satisfied until your next meal.

1½ cups unflavored plant-based protein powder

1 cup all-natural salted creamy peanut butter

1 cup honey

1 cup coconut flakes, for garnish (optional)

1. In a medium bowl, combine the protein powder, peanut butter, and honey. Stir until well combined into a stiff dough, about 2 minutes.
2. Using a spoon and your hands, divide and roll the dough into 20 (1- to 2-inch) balls.
3. If desired, pour the coconut flakes into a small bowl and roll each ball in the coconut to coat.
4. Store 2 balls per small airtight container or resealable bag in the refrigerator.

Substitution Tip: Whey-based protein powder can be used instead of plant-based. Vanilla or chocolate protein powder works great, too.

Per serving (2 balls): Calories: 317, Total fat: 14g, Total carbs: 35g, Sugar: 31g, Protein: 18g, Fiber: 2g, Sodium: 267mg

Raw Chocolate Chip Cookie Dough

CARDIO, DAIRY-FREE OPTION, NUT-FREE, VEGAN OPTION

PREP TIME: 15 MINUTES / **COOK TIME:** 10 MINUTES • **MAKES 6 SERVINGS**

Raw cookie dough is so delicious, but because of the uncooked eggs, it's not really safe to eat. This recipe has eliminated those risks to create a delicious edible dough. I've also modified the recipe to be a little healthier.

1 cup whole wheat pastry flour or all-purpose flour

¼ cup butter or coconut oil, at room temperature

2 tablespoons granulated sugar

½ cup packed brown sugar

½ teaspoon sea salt

3 tablespoons milk or plant-based alternative

1 teaspoon vanilla extract

¾ cup dark chocolate chips

1. Preheat the oven to 325°F.
2. Spread the flour on a baking sheet and bake for 10 minutes. (This sterilizes the flour.)
3. Allow the flour to cool for about 20 minutes.
4. In a medium bowl, mix together the butter, granulated sugar, and brown sugar until creamy, about 2 minutes.
5. Add the salt, milk, vanilla, and baked flour. Stir into a soft dough, about 2 minutes.
6. Stir in the chocolate chips.
7. Roll into 1- to 2-inch balls and evenly divide into small prep containers. Store in the refrigerator until needed.

Substitution Tip: Easily make this recipe vegan and dairy-free by using coconut oil and a plant-based milk.

Per serving (2 cookie balls): Calories: 367, Total fat: 18g, Total carbs: 48g, Sugar: 28g, Protein: 4g, Fiber: 5g, Sodium: 269mg

Pumpkin Walnut Cake

CARDIO, DAIRY-FREE, NUT-FREE OPTION, VEGAN OPTION

PREP TIME: 15 MINUTES / **COOK TIME:** 1 HOUR, PLUS 1 HOUR TO COOL • **MAKES 12 SERVINGS**

This dessert incorporates the goodness of pumpkin and walnuts to create a dessert that gives your body some good nutrition as well as a yummy treat. Pumpkin doesn't have to be just a fall dessert—it can be enjoyed all year long.

3 cups whole wheat flour
1 teaspoon sea salt
2 teaspoons baking powder
2 teaspoons baking soda
3½ teaspoons ground cinnamon
4 large eggs
1½ cups loosely packed brown sugar
¾ cup olive oil
1 (30-ounce) can pure pumpkin puree
1 cup chopped walnuts (optional)

1. Preheat the oven to 350°F. Line a 9-by-13-inch baking pan with parchment paper.
2. In a medium bowl, combine the flour, salt, baking powder, baking soda, and cinnamon and stir. Set aside.
3. In a large bowl, beat the eggs for 1 minute.
4. Add the brown sugar, oil, and pumpkin and whisk or beat well for about another minute.
5. Add the dry ingredients to the wet ingredients and mix gently for another minute.
6. Pour the batter into the prepared pan and sprinkle the walnuts (if using) evenly on top of the batter.
7. Bake for about 1 hour, or until a toothpick placed in the center comes out clean.
8. Allow to cool for 1 hour before cutting into 12 slices and storing in prep containers in the refrigerator.

Substitution Tip: This cake can be made vegan by swapping the eggs for 4 tablespoons of ground flaxseed and ¾ cup of water.

Per serving: Calories: 343, Total fat: 16g, Total carbs: 46g, Sugar: 20g, Protein: 7g, Fiber: 6g, Sodium: 518mg

Old-Fashioned Potato Candy

CARDIO, GLUTEN-FREE, VEGAN

PREP TIME: 15 MINUTES / **COOK TIME:** 6 MINUTES • **MAKES 20 PIECES**

This is a recipe my great-grandmother made, and it's been a family favorite for a long time. Using salted all-natural peanut butter adds some protein and healthy fats to this delicious and simple treat.

1 medium (4-inch) yellow potato
16 ounces confectioners' sugar
¾ cup salted creamy all-natural peanut butter

1. Wash the potato and puncture it with a fork on all sides. Cook the potato in the microwave for 3 minutes. Turn it over and cook for 3 more minutes.
2. Slice the potato in half and scoop out the cooked flesh into a medium bowl. Mash well with a fork or potato masher. Let cool until just slightly warm.
3. With a spoon or electric hand mixer, mix in the sugar, a little at a time, until a soft dough forms.
4. Form the dough into a log and place it on a 24-inch piece of parchment paper.
5. Use a rolling pin or glass, roll the dough lengthwise into a ¼-inch-thick rectangle.
6. Spread the peanut butter evenly over the dough. Roll the dough, starting at the end closest to you widthwise. Slice the roll into 20 equal pieces.
7. Store the potato candy in the refrigerator in small prep containers.

Ingredient Tip: This can be made with leftover mashed potatoes; use ½ cup with this option.

Per serving (2 pieces): Calories: 308, Total fat: 10g, Total carbs: 53g, Sugar: 47g, Protein: 5g, Fiber: 1g, Sodium: 85mg

No-Bake Peanut Butter and Chocolate Cookies

CARDIO, GLUTEN-FREE, STRENGTH/CARDIO, VEGETARIAN

PREP TIME: 5 MINUTES / **COOK TIME:** 10 MINUTES, PLUS 45 MINUTES TO COOL

MAKES 12 COOKIES

If you love peanut butter and chocolate, this easy cookie recipe will be right up your alley. Yes, these cookies have some sugar in them, but the oats, peanut butter, and cocoa provide wholesomeness, so it won't just be empty calories you're consuming with this treat.

4 tablespoons butter

2 tablespoons unsweetened cocoa powder

½ cup milk

1 cup sugar

1 teaspoon vanilla extract

3 cups quick-cook rolled oats

½ cup all-natural peanut butter

1. In a 2-quart pot over medium heat, melt the butter.
2. Stir in the cocoa powder until it is dissolved.
3. Add the milk and sugar, stirring constantly, and bring to a boil. Keep stirring the boiling mixture for 3 minutes.
4. Remove from the heat and stir in the vanilla, then the oats, then the peanut butter, making sure each ingredient is completely incorporated before adding the next one. Set aside.
5. Spread a 24-inch-long piece of parchment paper on your counter.
6. Drop tablespoon dollops of hot cookie mixture onto the parchment paper, giving them space to widen to 2 inches, until all the mixture has been used. You should have about 12 (2-inch) cookies.
7. Let cool for 30 to 45 minutes. Portion into resealable plastic bags and store on your counter for up to 1 week.

Prep Tip: Be sure to boil the full 3 minutes while stirring. This is what causes the cookies to firm up as they cool.

Per serving (2 cookies): Calories: 490, Total fat: 22g, Total carbs: 67g, Sugar: 36g, Protein: 12g, Fiber: 7g, Sodium: 75mg

Green Apple Cake

CARDIO, DAIRY-FREE, NUT-FREE, VEGETARIAN

PREP TIME: 10 MINUTES / **COOK TIME:** 40 MINUTES, PLUS 1 HOUR TO COOL • **MAKES 12 SERVINGS**

This apple cake uses real fruit to create a moist cake that doesn't need icing. In addition to apples, the grated carrots make this dessert sweet and nutritious. It's a dump-everything-in-and-mix type of recipe, so it's simple to make.

2 large eggs

1½ cups loosely packed brown sugar

½ cup olive oil

2 teaspoons ground cinnamon

1 teaspoon vanilla extract

2 cups whole wheat flour

½ teaspoon sea salt

2 teaspoons baking soda

2 carrots, grated

3 large or 4 medium Granny Smith apples, peeled, cored, and cut into ½-inch dice

1. Preheat the oven to 350°F. Line a 9-by-13-inch baking pan with parchment paper.
2. In a medium bowl, lightly beat the eggs.
3. Add the brown sugar, oil, cinnamon, vanilla, flour, salt, and baking soda and mix until combined, about 1 minute. Stir in the carrots and apples.
4. Using a rubber spatula, transfer the batter to the prepared baking pan and spread out evenly.
5. Bake for about 40 minutes, or until a toothpick placed in the center of the cake comes out clean.
6. Remove from the oven and let cool for 1 hour before cutting into 12 equal slices. Store in prep containers as needed.

Ingredient Tip: Granny Smith apples have a nice tart/sweet flavor and don't get mushy during baking, but any apples will work.

Substitution Tip: This cake can be made vegan by replacing the eggs with 2 tablespoons of ground flaxseed and 6 tablespoons of water.

Per serving: Calories: 263, Total fat: 10g, Total carbs: 41g, Sugar: 23g, Protein: 4g, Fiber: 4g, Sodium: 330mg

Banana Chia Overnight Pudding

CARDIO, GLUTEN-FREE, NUT-FREE, VEGAN

PREP TIME: 10 MINUTES • **MAKES 4 SERVINGS**

Chia seeds are really nutritious for their tiny size, but they also thicken liquids to create a creamy consistency without cooking. This recipe is a great way to use up overly ripe bananas. Because ripe bananas are pretty sweet already, no sugar is needed to make this healthy dessert.

4 ripe bananas
4 cups plant-based milk
2 tablespoons chia seeds
1 teaspoon vanilla extract

In a blender, combine the bananas, milk, chia seeds, and vanilla and blend on high for 1 minute. Evenly divide the pudding into each of 4 prep containers. Store in the refrigerator until needed.

Ingredient Tip: The chia will thicken as it sits in the refrigerator, but it needs at least one night.

Per serving: Calories: 192, Total fat: 5g, Total carbs: 38g, Sugar: 22g, Protein: 3g, Fiber: 6g, Sodium: 151mg

Blueberry Crumble

CARDIO, NUT-FREE, STRENGTH/CARDIO, VEGAN OPTION

PREP TIME: 10 MINUTES / **COOK TIME:** 40 MINUTES • **MAKES 6 SERVINGS**

This recipe incorporates high-antioxidant blueberries into a dessert that tastes like pie but is much easier to make and is healthier because of the whole grains. This crumble can be served cold or warm with vanilla ice cream or frozen yogurt.

4 cups frozen blueberries
1 cup whole wheat flour
2 cups quick-cook rolled oats
½ cup (1 stick) butter, at room temperature
½ teaspoon sea salt
¾ cup loosely packed brown sugar

1. Preheat the oven to 350°F. Line a 9-by-13-inch baking pan with parchment paper.
2. Spread the blueberries evenly in the pan.
3. In a medium bowl, combine the flour, oats, butter, salt, and brown sugar.
4. Mix until the butter has been incorporated into the dry ingredients and the mixture has a crumbly consistency. Sprinkle the "crumble" over the blueberries evenly.
5. Bake for about 40 minutes, or until the crumble is golden brown. Remove from the oven and let rest for 10 minutes.
6. Evenly divide the crumble into each of 6 prep containers. Store in the refrigerator until needed.

Reheat: From the refrigerator, with the lid cracked, heat in the microwave for 45 seconds.

Substitution Tip: This recipe can easily be made vegan by swapping the butter for an equal amount of coconut oil.

Per serving: Calories: 453, Total fat: 19g, Total carbs: 69g, Sugar: 31g, Protein: 7g, Fiber: 9g, Sodium: 327mg

Measurement Conversions

VOLUME EQUIVALENTS (LIQUID)

US STANDARD	US STANDARD (OUNCES)	METRIC (APPROXIMATE)
2 tablespoons	1 fl. oz.	30 mL
¼ cup	2 fl. oz.	60 mL
½ cup	4 fl. oz.	120 mL
1 cup	8 fl. oz.	240 mL
1½ cups	12 fl. oz.	355 mL
2 cups or 1 pint	16 fl. oz.	475 mL
4 cups or 1 quart	32 fl. oz.	1 L
1 gallon	128 fl. oz.	4 L

VOLUME EQUIVALENTS (DRY)

US STANDARD	METRIC (APPROXIMATE)
⅛ teaspoon	0.5 mL
¼ teaspoon	1 mL
½ teaspoon	2 mL
¾ teaspoon	4 mL
1 teaspoon	5 mL
1 tablespoon	15 mL
¼ cup	59 mL
⅓ cup	79 mL
½ cup	118 mL
⅔ cup	156 mL
¾ cup	177 mL
1 cup	235 mL
2 cups or 1 pint	475 mL
3 cups	700 mL
4 cups or 1 quart	1 L
½ gallon	2 L
1 gallon	4 L

WEIGHT EQUIVALENTS

US STANDARD	METRIC (APPROXIMATE)
½ ounce	15 g
1 ounce	30 g
2 ounces	60 g
4 ounces	115 g
8 ounces	225 g
12 ounces	340 g
16 ounces or 1 pound	455 g

OVEN TEMPERATURES

FAHRENHEIT (F)	CELSIUS (C) (APPROXIMATE)
250°	120°
300°	150°
325°	165°
350°	180°
375°	190°
400°	200°
425°	220°
450°	230°

Resources

Apps and calculators

Exercise Calorie Burn Calculator: HealthyEater.com/calories-burned

Food Nutrition Database: Fdc.nal.usda.gov

MapMyFitness App: MapMyFitness.com

MyFitnessPal App: MyFitnessPal.com

TDEE and Macro Calculator: HealthyEater.com/flexible-dieting-calculator

Books

Prep School: How to Improve Your Kitchen Skills and Cooking Techniques by James P. DeWan

References

"Calorie Restriction and Fasting Diets: What Do We Know?" 2021. *National Institute on Aging*. https://www.nia.nih.gov/health/calorie-restriction-and-fasting-diets-what-do-we-know.

"How Many Calories Michael Phelps Consumed as a Swimmer." OlympicTalk, NBC Sports, May 5, 2020. https://olympics.nbcsports.com/2020/05/05/michael-phelps-calories-swimming/.

Kelishadi, Roya. "Life-Cycle Approach for Prevention of Non Communicable Disease." *Primordial Prevention of Non Communicable Disease*. Springer, Cham, 2019. 1–6.

Kenney, W. Larry. "Dietary Water and Sodium Requirements for Active Adults." *Sports Sci* 17 (2004): 92.

Mifflin, M. D., S. T. St. Jeor, L. A. Hill, B. J. Scott, S. A. Daugherty, and Y. O. Koh. 1990. "A New Predictive Equation for Resting Energy Expenditure in Healthy Individuals." *The American Journal of Clinical Nutrition* 51 (2): 241–247. doi:10.1093/ajcn/51.2.241.

"Most People Consume Too Much Salt." 2021. *Centers for Disease Control and Prevention*. https://www.cdc.gov/salt/index.htm.

Schoenfeld, Brad Jon, and Alan Albert Aragon. "How Much Protein Can the Body Use in a Single Meal for Muscle-Building? Implications for Daily Protein Distribution." *Journal of the International Society of Sports Nutrition* 15, no. 1 (2018): 1–6.

"Trans Fat Is Double Trouble for Your Heart." 2021. Mayo Clinic. https://www.mayoclinic.org/diseases-conditions/high-blood-cholesterol/in-depth/trans-fat/art-20046114.

"Who Invented SMART Goals?" Reference.Com. https://www.reference.com/history/invented-smart-goals-91a96ac7407ac68a.

Index

C

D

E

F

G

H

J

L

M

N

Q

R

S

T

V

W

Y

Acknowledgments

I'd like to thank my mother for teaching me how to cook and not being afraid to let me make a mess in her kitchen when I was growing up. I'd also like to thank my husband for often being the guinea pig when I'm developing a new recipe for the first time. Lastly, I'd like to thank James Foster, who opened the door for me to start writing and blogging about diet and fitness more than 13 years ago. That door opened so many opportunities and possibilities, and I'll be forever grateful.

About the Author

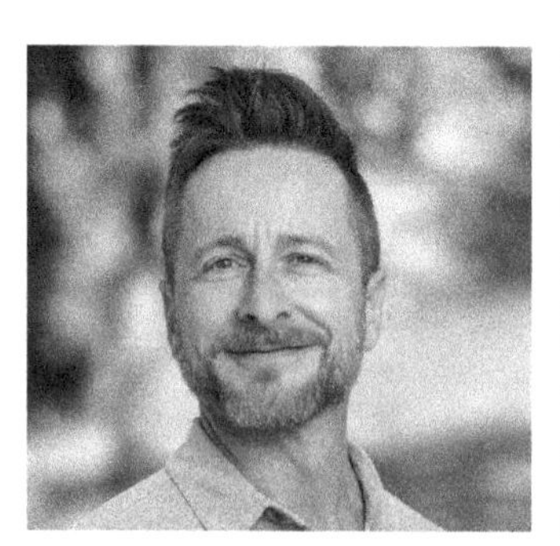

Ted Kallmyer, M.Ed., certified nutrition expert and coach, is the creator behind HealthyEater.com and the author of *The Macro Solution*. He loves to develop and cook healthy recipes for his family and friends and reinvent the Southern cooking he grew up on. His energized approach to weight loss and fitness coaching focuses on the unique needs of each client. He challenges them to feel exhilarated through discovering exciting new ways of eating healthy and still enjoying the foods they love, all the while achieving their fitness goals. Ted provides coaching services and resources through his website and is a sought-after media guest.

CPSIA information can be obtained
at www.ICGtesting.com
Printed in the USA
JSHW012319300122
22383JS00002B/3

9 781648 762925

THE HARMONY OF E
DEPENDENT-A

A COMMENTA
TSONGKHAPA'S

THE ESSENCE OF ELOQUENT SPEECH
PRAISE TO THE BUDDHA FOR TEACHING
PROFOUND DEPENDENT-ARISING

By

VEN. LOBSANG GYATSO

LIBRARY OF TIBETAN WORKS AND ARCHIVES

ISBN: 81-85102-83-X

Published by Library of Tibetan Works and Archives, Dharamsala, and printed at Indraprastha Press (CBT), 4 Bahadurshah Zafar Marg, New Delhi-110002.

CONTENTS

PUBLISHER'S NOTE

This work by Ven. Lobsang Gyatso titled "*The Harmony of Emptiness and Dependent-Arising*" is a commentary to Tsongkhapa's "*The Essence of Eloquent Speech, Praise to the Buddha for Teaching Profound Dependent-Arising.*" The subject matter of the work concerns two central themes of Buddhist philosophy - emptiness and dependent-arising.

All schools of Buddhism expound theories of emptiness and dependent-arising, but their interpretations vary greatly and are even contradictory. Here the author very skillfully explains the complementary nature of the different schools and gradually leads to the highest school of thought - Prasangika Madhyamika. All explanations are given through logical analysis combined with simple yet wonderful examples.

This work is a welcome contribution in that it is by a meditation master who is a man of great learning and who has many years of practical teaching experience. We hope that the readers will gain profound analytical insight into the view of dependent-arising and thus be able to to proceed their journey on the Mahayana path to the state of great enlightenment.

We would like to thank to Ven. Lobsang Gyatso for this valuable contribution not only in the study of emptiness and dependent-arising but on Buddhism as a whole. Our thanks also goes to Losang Chophel Ganchenpa for proof-reading the material and for his suggestions.

Gyatsho Tshering
Director, LTWA

March 1992

THE ROOT TEXT

THE ESSENCE OF ELOQUENT SPEECH
PRAISE TO THE BUDDHA FOR TEACHING
PROFOUND DEPENDENT-ARISING

(It is not known who made this translation of the primary text)

I bow down to him whose insight and speech
Make him unexcelled as sage and teacher;
The victor, who realised (ultimate truth),
Then taught us dependently-related arising.

Ignorance is the very root
Of all troubles in this transitory world.
These are averted by understanding
The dependent-arising which you have taught.

How then could the intelligent
Not understand that the path
Of dependently-related arising
Is the essence of your teaching?

This being so, O Saviour, who could find
Anything more wonderful
To praise you for
Than your teaching of the dependent-Arising?

Whatever depends on conditions
Is empty of inherent existence,
What excellent instruction could there be,
More amazing than these words?

Through wrongly holding (dependent-arising),
The childish strengthen bondage to extreme views.
But, for the wise, the same thing is the means
To cut free from the net of elaborations.

Since this teaching is not found elsewhere,
You alone are the 'Teacher.'
For a Tirthika, this name would be a flattery,
Like calling a fox a lion.

O wondrous teacher! O wondrous refuge!
Supreme speaker! Great protector!
I pay homage to the great teacher
Who so clearly explained dependent-arising.

O benefactor! To heal all beings
You proclaimed (dependent-arising),
The peerless reason for ascertaining
Emptiness, the heart of the teaching.

How could those who see the way
Of profound dependent-arising
As contradictory or unproven
Ever understand your system?

When one perceives 'empty'
As the meaning of 'dependent-arising,'
Empty of inherent existence does not contradict
The function of agent and action.

Whereas if one perceives the opposite,
Since there can be neither action in voidness
Nor emptiness in what has action,
One would fall into a dreadful abyss.

Therefore understanding dependent-arising,
As you have taught, is well praised.
(things) are not totally non-existent,
Nor are they inherently existent.

The independent is like a sky-flower.
Therefore, nothing is not dependent.
Existence with self-nature precludes
Establishment by causes and conditions.

Thus it is taught that because nothing exists
Other than the dependent-arisen,
There is no existing thing
Which is not empty of inherent existence.

Since inherent nature has no end, you said that
Nirvana would be impossible
If phenomena had any inherent nature,
For elaborations could not be stopped.

Therefore, who could challenge him
Who, in assemblies of the wise,
Has clearly proclaimed with lion's roar
Freedom from inherent nature?

Since lack of inherent nature,
And the ability to function do not contradict,
Never mind that dependent-arising
And emptiness co-exist.

'By the reason of dependent-arising,
There are no grounds for extreme views.'
For this fine teaching, O Protector,
Your speech is unexcelled.

'All is empty of self-nature!'
And, 'From this cause arises that effect!'
These two certainties assist each other
And abide in harmony.

What is more wonderful than this?
What is more marvelous than this?
If you are praised for this principle,
That is real praise; nothing else.

Those held in slavery by delusions,
Hopelessly resent you (so free and clear).
Small wonder that they find intolerable
That sound of, 'Non-inherent existence.'

But to accept dependent-arising,
The precious treasure of your speech,
Then resent the roar of emptiness;
This do I find surprising.

If through the very term of highest
Dependent-arising, the door that leads
To non-inherent existence they grasp
Inherent existence, by what means

Can these people be led into
The good path which pleases you,
That incomparable entrance,
Well travelled by supreme Aryas?

Inherent existence, unmade and non-dependent;
Dependent-related, made and dependent;
How can these two states be combined
On one base, without contradictions?

Therefore, whatever arises dependently
Though always free of inherent existence,
Appears to exist from its own side;
So you said this is like an illusion.

Through this very fact we cal well understand
The assertion that, in the way you taught.
Those who would challenge you
By way of logic can find no fallacy.

Why? Because your explanation
Make remote the chance that one
Will exaggerate or deny
Manifest or non-manifest things.

Your speech is seen as peerless
Because it presents the path of dependent-arising,
And this give rise to certainty
That (your) other teachings are valid too.

You saw reality, and taught it well.
Those who train in your footsteps
Will transcend all trouble,
For they shall destroy the root of evil.

But those who turn away from your teaching,
Though they wearily struggle, long and hard,
Invite problems, one after the other,
by their firm views of a self.

Marvellous! When the wise comprehend
The difference between these two (trainings),
How can they fail to respect you
From their innermost hearts?

Not to mention the entire wealth of your teachings
Just generally understanding
One small part of them,
Is to bring supreme bliss.

Alas! My own mind was ruled by confusion
When long ago I sought refuge,
Blind to your teachings' vast qualities,
Not to mention their fine details.

Yet the stream of life has not yet sunk
Into the mouth of the Lord of Death,
And I have a little belief in you.
Even this I think fortunate.

Of teachers, the teachers of dependent-arising.
Of wisdom, the wisdom of dependent-arising;
Like kings over all conquerors in the world,
These prove your wisdom supreme.

All that you have taught
Is related to dependent-arising;
And since this leads to Nirvana,
No deed of yours does not bring peace.

Wonderful is your teaching!
Since whoever listens
Will attain peace, who could not
Be devoted to preserving such teaching?

As it overcomes all opponents,
Is free from internal contradiction
And fulfills both goals of beings.
My delight ever grows for this Doctrine.

For the sake of the Doctrine, you gave
Again and again over countless aeons,
Sometimes your body, sometimes your life,
Your dear family, and treasures of wealth.

When I contemplate the excellences of your Dharma,
You appear to my mind
As a fish is drawn by the hook;
How said my fate to have not heard it from you.

The intensity of this sadness
Does not let my mind go free,
Just as a mother's mind never separates
From the thought of her beloved, lost child.

But when I reflect on your speech, thinking,
'Blazing with splendour of holy marks and signs,
Hallowed by rays of light,
O Teacher, with your beautiful Brahma voice,

You spoke in this way,' then in my mind
The image of Shakyamuni arises and
Immediately my sorrows are healed,
As moon beams soothe a fever.

Although this good system is so marvelous,
The unskilled become totally confused,
Ideas all tangled in every way,
Just like a balbaza grass.

Having understood the problem I then
Schooled myself (in the texts of) skilled sages,
And with energy listened here and there,
Ever seeking the meaning of your intention.

I studied many treatises
Of Buddhist and non-Buddhist schools,
Yet my mind was tormented sorely,
Time and again in the web of doubt.

Nagarjuna was prophesied to explain rightly
The principle of your final vehicle,
Free from the extremes of existence and non-existence.
When I, through the kindness of the lama,

Beheld the night-lily garden of his treatises
Illuminated by garlands of white light,
True eloquence of the glorious Moon (Chandrakirti),
Whose bright orb of immaculate wisdom

Moves freely across the sky of scripture,
Dispelling the darkness of extremist hearts
And outshining the constellations of wrong speech,
My mind found relief at last.

Of all his deeds, Buddha's speech is supreme,
And, for this very reason, true sages
Should commemorate the Perfect One
For this (teaching of dependent-arising).

Inspired by the Teacher, I renounced the world
And studied well the Conqueror's teaching,
I have been diligent in yoga practice - such is
This monk's reverence for the Great Seer.

By the kindness of my guru I was fortunate to meet
The liberating teaching of the peerless guide,
Therefore I dedicate this virtue as a cause
For all beings to be received by spiritual friends.

Until samsara ends, may the beneficent one's teaching
Be undisturbed by the winds of wrong views;
May all beings in the world forever understand
The essence of the teaching and have faith in the
teacher.

May they uphold Shakyamuni's excellent way,
Which reveals the principle of dependent-arising.
Through all their lives let them never waver,
Even at the cost of their bodies, or their lives.

Day and night may they always be thinking
How to best propagate this glorious success
Achieved by the Supreme Liberator, in lives
Of assiduous effort beyond measure.

When things strive with pure intention (to preserve this Doctrine),
May Brahma, Indra, the world's protectors
And the guardians, such as Mahakala,]
Be constant aides, never letting them down.

I

COMMENTARY

BY VEN LOBSANG GYATSO

VICTORIOUS

1

I bow down to him whose insight and speech
Make him unexcelled as sage and teacher,
The Victor who realized and taught
Dependently related arising.

Tsongkhapa, the author of *The Essence of Eloquent Speech, Praise to the Buddha for Teaching Profound Dependent-Arising* is renowned as one of the very greatest scholar-saints that Tibet has ever produced. He wrote this text on the morning that he abandoned all perplexities and wrong views and for the first time experienced direct insight into reality which is the essence of Buddha's wisdom. Tsongkhapa was born in 1357 in the Tsongkha district of Amdo province in north-east Tibet.[1] From a very early age his life was wholly devoted to the study and contemplation of the Buddha's words and he single-mindedly pursued the highest and most inspiring of goals, the complete enlightenment of a Buddha, in order to be able to help all other beings free themselves from suffering. After many years of receiving teachings, study, debate, contemplation and retreat, during which he himself became famous as a teacher, one night in 1398 he dreamed that he was present at a discussion of the intricacies of the ultimate view between the most illustrious Buddhist masters of the past. One, whose

---

[1] One of the sources for this paragraph on Tsong Khapa's biography is the introduction to *Tsong Khapa's Speech of Gold in the Essence of True Eloquence*, by Robert Thurman. Much greater detail will be found there.

commentary Tsongkhapa had been reading the previous evening, Buddhapalita, approached and blessed him by touching him on the head with a text. Thereupon Tsongkhapa awoke and turned again to Buddhapalita's commentary. As dawn was breaking he finally generated the blissful sun-like wisdom which experiences all things as they are and has the power to dispel forever the darkness of ignorance.

Praise for Dependent-Arising is Tsongkhapa's spontaneous outpouring of devotion to Shakyamuni Buddha for the unparalleled teachings which inspired and guided him through long years of practice and whose deepest truth he finally verified by his own direct realization on that morning. It is an expression of the author's redoubled faith in the Buddha, by its eloquence inspiring faith in others, drawing them into the study and practice of these teachings and setting them on the path which leads to the highest enlightenment. Tsongkhapa writes with a sense of fulfillment and precise certainty. With this assurance, his mind is turned completely towards benefitting all other beings in the world. If we could have an echo of this motivation in our minds as we read his verses and this commentary on them that would be excellent. Otherwise the contents of this book might become no more than a possible contribution to our general knowledge of the world. Reading to improve our general knowledge is fine, but when approaching *dharma* teachings ideally something more is called for. After all, the Sanskrit word *dharma* refers to instructions that hold us back from suffering. The Buddha showed how the cause of all the suffering we experience lies within, tracing it back to the deluded states of mind. Turbulent emotions such as jealousy, hatred, attachment and ignorant fanaticism are responsible for all harmful actions and consequent suffering. *Dharma* teachings are designed to nourish the mind, to bring about attitudes of equanimity and compassion so that we can remain happy whatever the external conditions. With the powerful sword of wisdom, we can sever the root of all other delusions which is ignorance. In doing so, we will achieve the state of complete liberation from suffering. Even the Buddha, whose knowledge is unlimited, was once a human being and began by relying on the encouragement and teachings of others in the way that is now open to us. So *dharma* teachings are not designed merely to be a pleasant diversion but to be a powerful medicine. If the teacher can teach and the student can listen, or read, in this spirit, putting far away all thoughts of fame, praise, material gain and mere worldly knowledge, great benefit can ensue.

Besides the work under consideration here, *The Essence of Eloquent Speech, Praise to the Buddha for Teaching Profound Dependent-Arising,* Tsongkhapa wrote another work, which has the words 'essence of eloquent speech' in the title. The full title of that great work is *The Essence of Eloquent Speech, Treatise Distinguishing the Interpretable and Definitive*. For this reason the verses we shall be discussing are sometimes known as the short *Essence of Eloquent Speech*, although we shall use the abbreviated title, *Praise for Dependent-Arising* in this book. The longer *Essence* presents a thorough evaluation of the different interpretations of the meaning of Buddha's deepest teachings that have been put forward by various Buddhist scholars and practitioners. *Praise for Dependent Arising,* as we shall see, a distillation of many of these points which affords an excellent introduction to the central philosophical issue of the Buddhist path to liberation, the equivalence of dependent-arising and emptiness.

In the first verse, Tsongkhapa, from all Buddha's good qualities, singles out his realization and teaching of dependently-related arising. The first verse is the expression of homage and Tsongkhapa bows low to the one whose insight makes him unsurpassed in wisdom. While other teachers teach from belief, from faith or teach wisdom that comes in the form of dogma, Buddha taught from a complete, direct understanding of his subject, and his theme is not something that will only be of temporary passing benefit to his listeners but is the wisdom which will release them completely from their burden of misunderstanding and misconception. Nor is there anyone besides the Buddha who taught dependent-arising so explicitly and so thoroughly, thus Buddha is unequalled in what he realized and what he taught. How he taught is also regarded as unequalled in that he had a special ability to teach in accordance with his listeners' predispositions and need. Through the completeness of his knowledge he understood the individual listeners' capacities and skillfully taught according to their level of understanding. This is reflected in the way Buddha's teachings came to be grouped in the Indian and Tibetan traditions. As we shall see, the teaching of dependent-arising has several different levels of interpretations, each particularly helpful for a certain type of person, but each superseded by a more refined and subtle presentation, until the Buddha's actual final view is arrived at.

The Buddha's teachings are not the kind of teachings that are merely attractive and pleasant to listen to, but they are able to bear reasoned analysis. This is perhaps the distinguishing feature of Buddha's teachings concerning the way to liberation. All religions present a path to a lasting kind of happiness, however it is called, but Buddha's path does not merely depend for its authenticity on revelation or on spiritual authority, nor is the resultant state of happiness bestowed by a ruling deity. Rather, freedom comes when we remove the defilements of ignorance from our own minds, first by verifying with our own wisdom the truth of dependent-arising and then by applying that wisdom in concentrated meditation. The Buddha has many marvellous qualities, and faith towards such a being will yield an abundance of good effects, but the best possible, most stable basis for such faith is not merely to believe out of awe and admiration that he teaches authentic path to eliminate suffering but to establish it with reasoning. In the texts on valid cognition, the great Buddhist logicians Dignaga and Dharmakirti do this by establishing the validity of the first teaching the Buddha gave after his enlightenment, the teaching on the four truths, which will be discussed below. The highest school of Buddhist philosophers, called the Middle Way Consequentialists, however, take Buddha's unique and unmistaken presentation of dependent-arising as their prime example of a valid teachings, for it is on the basis of the teaching of dependent-arising, conjoined with the view of emptiness that Buddha became the triumphant victor, as he is praise by Tsongkhapa in the first verse.

Buddha is a victor because he has finally, completely and irreversibly vanquished the two obscurations and the four maras. The two obscurations are the obscurations of delusion and the obscurations to knowledge. The first is the name given to the mental defilements or ignorance that prevent us from attaining personal liberation. The second is the name given to the defilements which obstruct our mind from attaining the unlimited direct understanding of a Buddha. 'Mara' means demon or evil spirit in Sanskrit but in a Buddhist context such hindering influences are regarded principally as aspects of our own imperfect condition rather than as externally existing foes. The first mara, for instance, is the mara of the aggregate. Our aggregates are the parts which make us up, basically our body and mind. Obviously there are many advantages to having the kind of body we have, but the term, mara of the aggregates, with reference to the body, covers all the shortcomings having such a body entails. Having such a body renders us vulnerable to a huge variety of sufferings, of hunger, thirst, heat, cold, illness, tiredness, aches, pains and injuries, despite our constant attempts to cherish and attend to its every whim. Since our aggregates cannot be dependent on and can hinder our progress in so many ways their unsatisfactory aspect is given the name mara.

The second of the maras is the mara of delusion, by which all negative states of mind such as anger, hatred, desirous attachment and pride are indicated. They are identified as a mara because they precipitate all harmful actions, from abusive speech to a mass murder. Not only that, when we are under the influence of a delusion it is most uncomfortable, such as when one boils with anger, and, unlike the suffering caused by external enemy which lasts for the maximum of one lifetime, the seeds of delusion, unless we do something about them, stay in our mind and accompany it from lifetime to lifetime. All forms of conflict can be traced back to this internal enemy, the conflicts between nations, between members of a family and right down to the fighting and arguing that goes on between small children.

The third mara, called the mara that is the son of a god, is something of an external troublemaker. As mentioned above, Buddhism identifies most causes of trouble as internal and shows that the remedy lies ultimately not in tinkering with the outside world but lies within. The mara, which is said to prey on beings who have a particularly strong resolve to achieve something positive, is something of an exception, but since it is also said to be dependent for its existence on people's superstition, the situation is not entirely cut and dried.

The last mara is the mara of death. Death is often personified as a particular being, the lord of death. This is a projection. What is intended here is the fact that we have to die soon enough, without knowing when and without the power to postpone it for a second. This great interrupter of life's hopes and aspirations is the fourth hinderance that Buddha is completely victorious over.

II

THE ROOT OF ALL TROUBLES

2

Ignorance is the very root
Of all troubles in this transitory world.
These are averted by understanding
The dependent-arising which you have taught.

All creatures are engaged in seeking happiness and trying to avoid suffering. Of those beings who are born with sufficient intelligence to be aware of their own motivation and have sufficient leisure to analyse what goals to aim at in life, many spend all their time in the pursuit of temporary forms of fulfillment, doubtful that there is any such thing as a permanent state of happiness, where suffering is completely abandoned. If pressed, these people may well admit that they suppose suffering, for instance in the form of old age, sickness and death, is ultimately inevitable and when such questions as, "Why are we here?" and, "Why is there dissatisfaction?" are posed their answer would be that, in these regions of investigation, man's lot is perplexity in the face of a mystery.

Those who have determinedly sought to penetrate this mystery have offered many paths of prayer and philosophy to the world, too many to be summarised properly here. There are those who have understood some aspects of the theory of *karma*, that we reap what we sow, in some form of future life if not in this, and make it their main practice to purify the seeds or potentials of bad actions they have previously committed by confession, prayer or by voluntary undergoing the hardship of physical penance. Others, tracing the origin of our problems back beyond the negative actions we have previously committed to the unwholesome conceptions that initiated them, principally endeavour to still the mind, to abandon all conception and eliminate discrimination as harmful in itself, in favour of some form of mental quietism. Others cultivate the practice of virtue. They practise generosity, patience and moral discipline. They live the life of love. The practice of benefitting others is most certainly supremely important, but thinking that that, by itself, is the whole path to the highest happiness in this or a future existence is mistaken, and the same applies to the other two types of practice we have mentioned. They are mistaken according to Tsongkhapa because, without understanding the profound dependent-arising, one cannot gain the ultimate view, without familiarising oneself again and again with the ultimate view, one cannot destroy ignorance; without destroying ignorance, one cannot find release from the sufferings of this transitory world, nor can one attain enormous beneficial potential of a fully enlightened being. Hence the utterly essential need to understand dependent-arising, set for in many different ways by the Buddha and condensed and celebrated here by Tsongkhapa.

We will thus be extremely fortunate if we can find a teacher who can explain dependent-arising to us flawlessly, for even within Buddhist philosophy there are a variety of different treatments of this central issue. Our way to proceed will be by bringing together the teachings of living master or masters, and our own analysis and study of the Buddhist texts. There are four Buddhist schools, called the Particularists, the Sutra-followers, the Proponents of Mind Only and the Proponents of the Middle Way. The last school has two divisions, the

Autonomists and the Consequentialists.[2] The explanation of dependent-arising reaches its fullest power in the commentaries of the Consequentialists whose foremost exponent in the Land of Snow was Tsongkhapa. Briefly at this stage, the schools of Mind Only and below only understand dependent-arising in terms of effects dependent on their causes, taking no account of uncaused or permanent i.e. unchanging phenomena. The Middle Way Autonomists extend the meaning of dependent-arising by showing how all phenomena, caused and uncaused, exits within the nature of dependent-arising, in the sense that they depend on their parts. For instance, a pot is not self-powered; it depends for its existence on its causes. Also it depends on its parts because without perceiving the parts of a pot, one cannot perceive a pot. The Consequentialists accept the above viewpoints but add various perspectives of their own, arguing that cause and effect are mutually dependent, as are self and other, and further reinterpret all other forms of dependent relationship in the light of their being dependent arisen

---

[2] The Sanskrit and Tibetan names of the followers of the various Buddhist schools are as follows:

English	Sanskrit	Tibetan
Particularist	Vaibhashika	bye brag smra ba
Sutra-follower	Sautrantika	mdo sde pa
Proponents of Mind Only	Chittamatra	sems tsam pa
Proponents of the Middle Way	Madhyamika	dbu ma pa
Autonomist	Svatantrika	rang rgyud pa
Consequentialist	Prasangika	thal 'gyur pa

in the sense of being mere imputations, upon a basis of designation, by a designating consciousness.

The above brief review of dependent-arising, various manifestations in the various schools of Buddhism maps out part of the route our investigation will take in later chapters. However, before we discuss how to cultivate the wisdom understanding dependent-arising, the antidote which will eliminate all our suffering, we first have to justify the diagnosis that ignorance is the primary cause of the disease, 'The root of all troubles in this transitory world.' First we will base our investigation on the teaching of the four truths and second on the teaching of twelve links of dependent-arising.

THE FOUR TRUTHS

If someone is ill, in order to treat the person and make him well, the doctor first has to take careful note of the symptoms of the disease and from them determine its root causes. Just administering medicine to relieve the symptoms will not do; the patient wants a remedy that will cure the disease completely and bring him to sound health. Having made his diagnosis, the doctor then prescribes a course of treatment appropriate to the disease which is designed to get rid of it. Finally the patient follows the doctor's instructions and is cured. This analogy serves well to introduce the four truths and their sequence. According to the analogy we are the patients and our condition is known as true suffering, which is the first of the truths. True suffering refers to all the trouble we face, all the forms of pain and dissatisfaction we encounter in this round of existence. However exalted our worldly status, we have to endure physical pain and mental anxiety. We do not escape the pangs of birth, aging, sickness and death. We never seem to be satisfied; we may have what we need, but we always crave for more. If we get what we desire, after enjoying it for a while we start to hanker after something else. If we do feel we are happy at a certain moment, we have to acknowledge the unsatisfactory feeling that, in the nature of things, we are bound to undergo suffering again, sooner or later.

The troubles of this world are easy to enumerate at length. Searching for their ultimate source, like the doctor trying to determine the root cause of the patient's illness, is more of a challenge. The causes of true sufferings are what are known as true origins, the second of the four truths. There are two divisions of true origins, *karma*, or action, and delusion. The first, *karma*, arises in dependence on the second, delusion. Delusions are various, attachment, hatred, pride, envy and so forth, the ultimate source of them all being, as Tsongkhapa says, ignorance. This, the second of the four truths is the one we are going to dwell on in this presentation of the four. In outline, the third truth is true cessation. It is synonymous with liberation, the final abandonment of suffering. In our medical analogy it is equivalent to the state of good health the sick person wishes to achieve. In other words it refers to the goal of religious practice or philosophy. The fourth truth is true paths. True paths refers to the realisations which are the antidote to the ignorance which is identified as true origins. They are thus like treatment prescribed by the doctor once he has properly identified his patient's illness. Those who have gone to liberation did so by generating these realisations in their minds.

Returning to the second truth, true origins, how ignorance is responsible for all the problems we encounter can be illustrated with the example of the effects of killing. The ignorance in questions, the ignorance concerning dependent-arising has two main aspects, ignorance of *karma* and ignorance of the ultimate nature of phenomena. The ignorance concerning the workings of *karma* will be described first.

There are those who actually enjoy killing, such as a hunter or fisherman who regard killing as sport. There are butchers too, who enjoy killing and do it with enthusiasm, thinking of the profit they will obtain from selling the meat of their victims. To such a one the effect of the killing is happiness; he deliberately engages in the action in the expectation of pleasure. It may well be that in the short term his expectations are fulfilled; the hunter enjoys his meal or his stuffed trophy and the butcher his profits. The long term effects of their actions are, however, far from being pleasurable, according to the principles of *karma*, the first of which states that actions are never wasted; they are certain to produce similar consequences, possibly in this life; usually in future lives.[3] Those who take life will experience suffering proportionate to the suffering they inflicted and the degree of enthusiasm with which they inflicted it. One who commits very harmful actions is liable to take rebirth in a lower state of existence, hellish or ghostly

---

[3] The Buddhist world view acknowledges the primacy of mind. In this view mind cannot arise out of a conglomeration of insensible material particles, during the process of embryonic development for instance. An individual's mind has experienced many previous lives before inhabiting the present body and the process of rebirth will go on until liberation is achieved.

for instance, or if the action is less intensely negative, he may take an animal rebirth. Other consequences may also flow from his act of killing. Even if he is born in a higher realm, his life span may be very short and he may have the inclination or tendency to enjoy taking life again and again. On the other hand there is always the possibility of purifying negative *karma* through the appropriate *dharma* practices in which case none of the above consequences are absolutely certain to occur. Much too depends on the strength of motivation. In our example we painted a picture of a very strong negative motivation which would incline those beings to be born in a hellish existence, but one can kill accidentally and it is not altogether impossible to kill with a virtuous motivation, free of self-cherishing. In these circumstances, the negative action of killing would still be committed but the ripened effects of the action would no doubt be lighter. The way the ripened effects of different actions can blend together is another variable. Here we are referring to what are known as projecting *karma* and completing *karma*. The projecting *karma* from an act of killing might for instance project or throw us into a lower state of existence, such as being born as a dog. Then completing *karma* deriving from a previous positive action might ripen during that life as a dog such that we are sheltered by kind people who provide us with excellent food and other comforts. Similarly, good projecting *karma* can bring about a higher state of rebirth only for it to be complemented by miserable completing *karma*.

Basically, all the pleasure we experience comes about due to our having committed virtuous actions, actions which benefit others, and all the suffering we experience comes about due to our having accumulated non-virtuous or harmful actions. The butcher of our example does not understand the true nature of the situations and he grasps that the action of killing will bring him pleasure and profit. Neither knowing nor caring about the long-term effects of his actions, snatching at the temporary pleasures of this life and indulging in the negative passions of greed and self-cherishing, he is whirled again and again into the troubles of this transitory round of existence, a leaf blown by the wind of his *karma* or past actions.

It is crucial for us to contemplate this facet of dependent-arising very carefully and gain conviction concerning the principles of *karma*. One who does can then determine firmly to abandon the taking of life. The firmer the decision the better; there is a much stronger beneficial effect from not killing having actively determined not to do so than from merely happening not to kill. The former is an actual wholesome or virtuous action whose effect will be happiness possibly leading to a future rebirth in one of the higher realms, as a human with a spark of intelligence, or amongst the gods who enjoy again and again the pleasures of refined sense gratification or the bliss of exalted states of meditative stabilization. But even those who are born in these worldly divine realms have not escaped suffering for good. They have not overcome the mara of death, for instance. In due course their happiness will come to an end. They will experience the trauma of death and rebirth again and migrate to another life, and yet another. A person who is still ensnared by false notions of the self, the root cause of suffering, and is ignorant of the power of the antidote, meditation on dependent-arising and selflessness, although he may have a correct understanding of *karma* which leads him to abandon killing, he has not entirely overcome the mara of delusion. His desires still remain focused on cyclic existence.

By contrast there is the person who, with the additional guidance of some understanding of the ultimate nature of the self, develops a pure and powerful wish to take control and free himself from the whole unsatisfactory round of death and rebirth powered by delusion and unskillful action. The clarity of the insight that Tsongkhapa attained on the morning that he composed this praise is such that the ignorance which throws us again and again into misery cannot abide simultaneously with it, no more than heat and cold can exist on the same spot. The ignorance is forced to give way just as the darkness in a room vanishes when we turn on the light. For somebody who has recognized the power of such wisdom and has thereby generated an authentic determination to emerge from cyclic existence, the effects of his action of decisively refraining from killing are in accordance with this strong wish and lead not to further involvement in the world but out of it, to liberation.

Abandoning killing in the hope gaining release from cyclic existence is still not the highest motivation we can aspire to. We abandon killing and experience some form of pleasure within cyclic existence. Beyond that we can abandon killing as part of our efforts to gain our own individual liberation from it, but best of all is to abandon killing with the pure wish to be of the utmost benefit to as many sentient beings as possible. One dwells on the fact that sufferings descend on all creatures alike, not just on oneself, and contemplates that a Buddha is the one who has the highest wisdom and most skilful means to separate being from their sufferings. Then one develops the spontaneous resolve to become a Buddha oneself for the benefit of all. This is called bodhicitta or the mind of enlightenment. When coupled with the precious bodhicitta in this way, the virtuous action of abandoning killing contributes to our own achievement of Buddhahood. Buddhahood is the highest enlightenment because it is for the sake not of oneself alone but for all sentient beings.

Depending on our motivation then, the long-term results of our virtuous actions such as avoiding harming others or generosity can either be worldly pleasure, the happiness of individual liberation or the fulfillment of complete enlightenment. Whether we can develop the more worthwhile second or third levels of motivation depends on whether our minds are obscured or not with regard to the ultimate nature of the self and phenomena. If it is, then the effects of all our actions, whether virtuous or non-virtuous, will ripen as further experiences within cyclic existence. In this sense our ignorance can be called the creator of the world. The Indian Middle Way master Aryadeva said in *The Four Hundred*,

> Ignorance pervades all delusions,
> Just as the physical sense faculty resides throughout the body.
> Thus when ignorance is destroyed,
> All other delusions will be destroyed too.

On the other hand, the wisdom which dispels such ignorance, the wisdom understanding ultimate nature, which is generated from our understanding of dependent-arising, is said to be the creator of the states of liberation and enlightenment. Some Buddhist schools in fact say that *karma* is the creator of the world. The highest school, the Consequentialists say that it is the mind or ignorance. These explanations are not contradictory. To give an analogy, *karma* can be likened to the soldiers who perform the acts of shooting and killing in a battle, while ignorance can be likened to the president of a country who orders his troops to war. We can point out fingers at the soldiers and say they did the killing but equally we can say that the ultimate responsibility for those acts lies with the president. In any case, when tracing back to the ultimate cause of the world, Buddhist thought goes back no further than our own minds. Buddhist thinkers have found no place for a creator-being, an architect or prime mover who of his own volition brings forth the universe. The source of our problems lies within our own minds, and so does the remedy. This is the import of the Buddha's teaching of the four truths.

TWELVE LINKS OF DEPENDENT-ARISING

A brief reference to another of the Buddha's teachings, the twelve links of dependent-arising, should further open the way to understanding the benefits of realizing dependent-arising that Tsongkhapa celebrates in this praise. We will recognize these benefits when we understand more clearly about the nature of cyclic existence. Cyclic existence refers to life in those worlds or realms, such as ours in which suffering occurs. Every state within it is transient and unstable. It is characterized as round because we are born here again and again. We are bound to wheel of existence because our births here are under compulsion and the cycle is very difficult to get rid of. The twelve links of dependent-arising are often drawn or painted in the form a wheel, held fast in the embrace of *Shinje*, the Lord of Death. The twelve links are (1) ignorance; (2) compounded *karma*; (3) consciousness; (4) name and form; (5) six sources; (6) contact; (7) feeling; (8) desirous attachment; (9) grasping; (10) existence; (11) birth; (12) aging and death.

The first of the twelve links is ignorance, and the root ignorance is ignorance concerning the ultimate nature of phenomena. Under the influence of this ignorance, a person commits an action, whether positive, negative or neutral, and this action forms the second link, compounded *karma*. Until it ripens in a future lifetime or later in this one, this action is, as it were, stored in the consciousness in the form of a potential or seed. Consciousness is the third link, and it is like the earth in which a seed rests until the other conditions necessary for it to germinate come together. If a seed is to germinate, one condition it certainly needs is moisture. In the case of the karmic seed, the equivalent of moisture is desirous attachment, attachment to the forms and features of cyclic existence with which one has such an ingrained familiarity. In the sequence of twelve links, attachment is placed eighth, but it is to that one we must now jump in this condensed explanation of the twelve links in terms of two lifetimes. The attachment particularly referred to here is the attachment to some feature of cyclic existence that manifests in the mind of someone who is on the verge of death. The next link, the ninth, grasping, is when that attachment strengthens up. As a person's gross sense consciousness shut down at death, there arises a strong inclination for a particular type of rebirth, as a certain kind of animal, as a human, a god or whatever. Appearances are said to arise to the mind of the forms or birth places the mind is attracted towards and will be associated with. The tenth link is called existence and refers to that fully potentialized *karma*, or action, which throws a person into a new life. The action of the second link has now ripened up, now all the conditions, such as attachment have come together. The six links we have mentioned so far, the first, second, third, eighth, ninth and tenth are, in this presentation, a causal sequence and the link of existence is the last moment of that sequence. The relationship between the body and mind of the person in that particular life now ceases. The consciousness departs from one life and goes on to the next.

The next link in the twelve, the first of the effect sequence, is birth, although between the end of one life and the start of another there is an intermediate stage. In this in-between state one has a body but is such a subtle type of form that it is not obstructed by gross matter such as walls and so forth, and it is not visible to ordinary eyes, although it is said to bear some resemblance to the form of the type of being one will become in the next life. We can think of radio broadcast being transmitted from the radio station to the place where someone is listening to the radio. Something travels from the broadcasting station to the receiver. It is not sound. We could say it is the potential to produce sound. The force which causes the radio waves to travel from one place to another in our illustration is like the fully potentialized *karma* in terms of the twelve links. When the sound waves reach a receiver, various sounds come forth. Similarly the force of *karma* propels a consciousness together with its very subtle energy body to a new place of birth where it unites with a new body of gross form, the joining sperm and egg of the mother and father in the case of human and most animal births, and rises as a new creature. Strictly speaking, however, the link of birth begins with the adoption of the body of the intermediate state right after death.

Of all the actions we have done whose effects have not yet worked themselves out, only one, the one ripening just at death, is responsible for determining what broad kind of rebirth we will experience. Why should one particular action, and not another, ripen up at this crucial time? Some actions leave a trace on the mind that is too weak ever to ripen up. Some actions are more liable to ripen up because the impression they left on the mind was sharp and strong. There is also the factor of how familiar we are with a certain action. The more familiar we are with a particular action, the more likely it is that it will be the strongest at the moment of death and the one that steers us to our new world. Can the consciousness and body separate other than at the time death? Yes, this can occasionally happen. There is a type of separation, if not a complete one, that can occur in sleep. There are also special techniques of meditation and concentration that enable an adept deliberately to separate the two, but for most people, when their mind and body come apart, it means they have reached the end of their life.

To continue with our enumeration of the twelve links, from birth, the eleventh link, we shift to the link of name and form, the fourth on the wheel of twelve and the second of the effect links. The link of name and form begins when the consciousness joins with its new form or body. After this comes the stage at which the same powers (five physical and one mental) arise in the unborn creature. This is called the link of the six sources.[4] The six sources are the fifth link and contact is the sixth. With the stage of contact the sense consciousness, the eye consciousness, the ear consciousness and so forth, start to have involvement with their objects. The subtle consciousness which entered the womb has given rise to gross levels of consciousness once more and these have their avenues of communication, the sense powers. They make contact with their objects and then the seventh link, feeling, occurs. All the while the process of aging has been going on and death has been approaching. Aging and death constitute the twelfth and final link. Another circuit of the wheel of existence comes to an end when the twelfth link's second stage, death, is complete. When life cannot be prolonged any further, the gross consciousness dissolve back into the subtle, the mind leaves its old body and heads towards the next life.

In terms of this present life, in the life prior to this one, we created the first three links, ignorance, compounded *karma* and consciousness, and also links eight, nine and ten: desirous attachment, grasping and existence. These are the six causal links which brought about this life. The remaining six links: four, name and form; five, six sources; six, contact; seven, feeling; eleven, birth; twelve, aging and death are the six effect links

---

[4] The five physical sense powers are not identified as the sense organs themselves but as a kind of clear form located within them. They give to their respective consciousness the ability to apprehend and to be generated in the aspect of their respective objects. The sixth sense power, which empowers mental as opposed to sense consciousness, is not physical, but is a previous moment of consciousness. For further details see *Meditation on Emptiness* by Jeffrey Hopkins.

which we are now passing through in this life. Only the final portion of the final link, death, has not been completed yet. Of course we are accumulating many different actions all the time. Any of these actions that are strong enough can give rise to a future birth, be it in a human realm, an animal realm, a hell realm or any other realm. We are continually creating causes for being reborn again. Even now, while we are experiencing the six effect links as we have just indicated, we are also going through the six causal links that will culminate in the next life. It is impossible to point a finger and say, 'This is the start of it all.' This beginningless round is what is referred to by the term cyclic existence or samsara. It is a process of continually creating *karma* and being reborn. All the four Buddhist schools we named earlier accept the description of the round of existence contained within the teaching on the twelve links of dependent-arising and the four truths. We should meditate upon it repeatedly in order to generate the mind determined to emerge from it. If we do, we will be drawn again and again to probe the ignorance that is 'the very root of all troubles in this transitory world,' and to wonder just what is the understanding of dependent-arising which shatters it asunder.

We have already noted that these verses are a spontaneous expression of Tsongkhapa's gratitude to the teacher Shakyamuni Buddha composed on the morning that he first gained a pure direct realization of the highest Buddhist view. All wrong views cast aside and inspired by the deepest faith, he prostrates and offers praises to Buddha, thus adding to the great wave of positive or meritorious energy that will carry him to the state of highest enlightenment. The poem will only achieve its complete purpose, however, if many of us too have our admiration awakened for a noble teacher and his penetrating teachings, and have a strength of conviction that will carry us through our studies, at least to the point where we become fully convinced of the validity of the endeavour and the worthiness of attaining the goals, individual liberation or fully enlightenment.

3

How then could the intelligent
Not understand that the path
Of dependently related arising
Is the essence of your teaching?

4

This being so, O Saviour
Who could find anything
More wonderful to praise you for
Than your teaching of dependent-arising?

While we contemplate the disadvantages of all states of rebirth in the cyclic existence in order to turn away from its superficial allurements, we should exert effort in thinking about the advantages of the peaceful state of liberation in order to make the wish to go there our strongest urge. The mind which understands dependent-arising is itself the path of verse three. A path we generally understand as a way we walk along to get to a certain destination. In the present context it is apt to call the mind which realizes dependent-arising a path because, once we have cultivated it, familiarising again and again on it, dwelling on that mind in meditation, is the way we travel to liberation. Dependent-arising is thus the essence of the teaching because realization of it is the key to becoming free from cyclic existence and going to enlightenment, as those who have turned their minds away from cyclic existence and have gained an understanding of dependent-arising, 'the intelligent,' surely know. This is why Tsongkhapa praises Shakyamuni Buddha above all for this wonderful gift of teachings on this topic. While other philosophers and practitioners pursue the same goal of highest happiness, of the hosts of teachers and guides, only the Buddha reveals the technique of dependent-arising, unsurpassed in effectiveness, and of the Buddhist schools, only the Consequentialists are able to explain it in all its magnificent depth and clarity. To do justice to the profundity of Tsongkhapa's verses, it is to an illumination of these assertions that we must now proceed, beginning with the views of the other schools, Buddhist and non-Buddhist, that Consequentialists either refute or surpass.

III

CAUSE AND EFFECT

5ab

Whatever depends on causes and conditions
Is empty of inherent existence.

Consider first how we ordinarily grasp things to exist. Do we not feel that the self and the everyday objects around us are established from their own side, that 'I' and the objects I use and possess are each substantial, solid, 'concretely pointoutable' entities? We can experience a sense of ourselves existing from our own side very vividly when we are in a perilous situation such as when we go to too near the edge of a steep cliff. At that time do we not appear to ourselves to exist by our own power, solidly and independently, having a nature that exists from within ourselves? But all our everyday perceptions are also tinged with this type of grasping. When we glance at our watch, for example, does it not appear to have its own independent, self-sufficient nature over and above any relationship that may be said to exist between it and other phenomena?

The Middle Way Consequentialists argue that all phenomena arise in dependence on causes and conditions and are therefore not established from their own side, do not exist by way of their own entity and are not inherently existent. Understanding this thoroughly is the way to remove the troubles of this transitory world. Apart from the Consequentialists, however, most schools of thought, Buddhist and non-Buddhist, western and eastern assume that phenomena do exist inherently, in the way that they appear.

Christians accept that the world was created by God, while God's existence on the other hand is not under the influence of causes and conditions. If the creation of

God is discussed at all the answer would seem to be that he is eternal or self-created. Many Hindu traditions adopt a similar point of view, crediting the creation of the world to a deity, Ishvara, who himself is unaffected by causes and conditions and who abides beyond fluctuation and instability. So both Christian and Hindu philosophers point to cause and effect relationships when trying to explain how things came about and how they exists. Tracing the causes backwards they arrive at a primordial being who stand outside the realm of change, an ultimate source from which all other phenomena derive their truly or inherently existent natures. The Hindu schools who accept rebirth view the 'I' or 'self' in a similar fashion. According to their reasoning we observe ourselves working, reading, eating and so forth. Then, tracing all these actions back to their source, we arrive at the self. It is the 'I' which causes all these actions to be performed. The source of our actions, they argue, has to be something substantial, truly existent, even unchanging. If the 'I' is forever changing, they say, how can we speak of an 'I' that goes from one life to another?

However, if we look into the implications of these assertions, for instance that there is such a thing as a creator deity who does not change, or that the 'I' is permanent or unchanging, we will find that they create rather more problems than they solve. Are not God before the creation of the universe and God who has created the universe necessarily different? And is it not a case of the former changing into the latter, in the same way that a childless woman has to change in some way in order to become a mother? A God that is beyond change and a God that is the creator of the universe are therefore incompatible. The idea of an unchanging 'I' is similarly problematic. Unfortunately there are many intelligent people these days who have come across one or two defective systems of thought and have identified many faults. This has discouraged them and led them to forsake the study and practice of religion and philosophy entirely.

A world view very familiar to Westerners who are coming into contact with Buddhist ideas these days is that formed under the influence of scientific discoveries and techniques of investigation, so a few comparative remarks about science and Buddhism may not be amiss for Westerns approaching the topic of dependent-arising. In their practical application Buddhism and science may be strikingly different, but in terms of view there are many explanations where the two systems are in accord, differing in emphasis rather than in fundamentals. Whereas science has been most successful in uncovering the workings of external phenomena such as matter, Buddhism's focus has always been on internal phenomena, namely on the mind. Obviously scientific investigation has revealed things that Buddhism has not touched upon and vice versa but it would be difficult to point to a subject where the two systems' assertions actually clash. This gives grounds for supposing that as research and investigation continue the two ways of thought could come closer together.

If we compare the theories of the origin of the universe and its contents presented in the scientific and Buddhist traditions a similar view of the process emerges. Various explanations of how this world, the other planets and the stars originated are put forward in different scientific theories, a common theme of which seems to be that though a beginning can be posited for the various heavenly bodies and so forth, the process of becoming in the universe in general is not something which scientists can state had a particular beginning. Whatever phenomena they trace back to, itself in turn must have had a cause. Down on the atomic level we find the same broad conclusion obtaining. Many minute particles temporarily conglomerate to form a material object which then in the fullness of time disintegrates. Individual gross forms arise and fall apart or are destroyed, but it is not possible to posit a beginning to the process. Any atomic substance or element has to have a cause. That cause must also have a cause and so on. Buddhist scholars have no quarrel with all this; rather they extend this understanding to the mind. Just as it seems simplest to say that matter has always been around in one manifestation or another so, we say, has mind, basically for the same reasons.

The scientific description of the conception and development of a child in the womb deals principally with the manifest physical aspects, from the meeting of the sperm and ovum onwards, whereas the Buddhists, while not faulting this explanation, bring three other elements to the fore, consciousness, subtle form and *karma*. A consciousness which has some time previously separated from its former body, and which contains the karmic seeds or potentials deposited on it by previous actions, together with its support, a very subtle kind of form, enters the womb at the time of conception and joins with the uniting sperm and ovum, its new body. As the child grows in the womb, science can furnish a very accurate picture of the different stages of its physical development. The Buddhist texts speak more about the inner experience of the child during this time. Again, these two versions of the first stage of life would seem to be quite compatible. The points of view are different but there is nothing in the Buddhist description which contradicts the scientific one and the Buddhist finds the scientific description complementary to his own.

Mind is in essence clear and cognizing. The only thing which can become the entity of the present moment of any individual's mind–and this includes the mind of an individual at the first moment of conception–is the previous moment of that mind. How can something which does not have the qualities of being clear and knowing and does not experience happiness and sorrow change into something which is clear and knowing and does experience happiness and sorrow? Matter cannot be produced in the entity of something clear and cognizing. Each individual's mind is a non-material phenomena which does not have any beginning; nor does it have any end. Everyone's stream of consciousness is constantly changing. Sometimes such a stream of consciousness takes a gross form, the ordinary sense consciousness being considered gross. Sometimes it takes a subtle form, for instance during the death process. Sometimes the delusions such as anger, hatred and pride flare up. Sometimes they are not manifest, existing only as potentials. The influence of ignorance is always present to some degree in an ordinary person's consciousness; affecting every cognition such a person has. Associated with every consciousness and acting as its basis is a very subtle kind of form or energy called subtle wind. Like the mind it accompanies, it cannot be said to have any beginning. Nor indeed can we who, as it were, possess our particular stream of consciousness be said, in a sense, to have any beginning. A person in this sense of the world goes from life to life, sometimes being born in the human realm, sometimes being born as animal or else as a god or some other creature. The gross physical forms are adopted and discarded while the consciousness migrates on and on from one existence to another. Upon death, anyone who has not mentally evolved to the point where he or she can step off this round will be thrust yet again into an existence where suffering occurs.

The main goal of *dharma* practice is to bring to an end the process of uncontrolled rebirth because what it amounts to is suffering. The means lies in our capacity for mental evolution. Hence the main subject for analysis and investigation in Buddhist philosophy is the mind. If we briefly mention one or two of the major classifications of mind in the Buddhist system there is first of all the division into two, valid and non-valid awarenesses, those that correctly apprehend a particular aspect of reality and induce certainty with respect to it and those that do not.[5] A careful study of these two types of mind is most worthwhile. For instance, an investigation of valid minds reveals two distinct kinds, direct valid perceivers and inferential valid cognizers. Some of the key objects of contemplation and meditation on the path to liberation such as emptiness and dependent-arising are quite subtle affairs so an ordinary being cannot observe them by direct perception, though that is his eventual aim. To understand them in the beginning he has to depend on an inferential

---

[5] We noted earlier that in an ordinary person's continuum every one of his cognitions is affected by ignorance. But the fact an ordinary person's valid awareness is not totally free of the effects of ignorance does not mean that it cannot be correct with respect to the main features of its object. For instance, we can still see and recognize a friend when we are wearing dark glasses which prevents us from seeing colours properly.

cognition which is basically the type of infallible mind which relies on a reason. To give a simple example of an inferential cognition: suppose we are standing outside a house and we see smoke rising from the chimney. In dependence on cognizing smoke we can infer that there is fire combustion inside the house. We cannot see the fire directly but we can have accurate knowledge of it by relying on a correct sign, smoke. The first type of wisdom that we cultivate to guide us on the path to liberation will be of this type which depends on reasons, so a particularly carefully study of this kind of mind is found in the Buddhist texts. The exactness, thoroughness and helpfulness of the Buddhist treatises on psychology could easily be illustrated with many examples but perhaps enough has been said now to plant the suggestion that just as science has evolved its own appropriate method of experimentation and investigation and has made countless discoveries, mainly concerning the external world, just so has Buddhism adopted and developed the techniques of analysis and reasoning, to say nothing of concentration and mediation, to its own purpose of formulating the laws by which the mind operates, to provide the basis for our step by step evolution to the highest states of happiness.

Considering now how cause and effect relationships are interpreted within the Buddhist schools, we find two contradictory views. In the quotation from the *Praise for Dependent-Arising* at the beginning of this chapter Tsongkhapa sets forth the view of dependent-arising that is exclusive to the Consequentialist schools. In contrast, the lower Buddhist schools adopt quite the opposite stance and argue that the fact that something arises in dependence on causes and conditions actually establishes that it *is* inherently existent. The lower schools detect no discrepancy between the appearance of phenomena as inherently existent and their actual mode of existence. When all is said and done, some of them would argue, we can see with our eyes that things are inherently existent. If we refuse to accept our own bare sense perceptions as valid, how can we possibly discriminate between what exists and what does not? We have no choice but to say that our sense perceptions are by and large in direct contact with reality. Things like cups, houses and table which appear to our senses to exist by way of their own independent entities really exist in that way. Certainly such things are created from cause and conditions but could they really exist if they did not have independent entities? Nagarjuna, a great Indian commentator who pioneered the Middle Way School of interpretation and brought what are known as the Great Vehicle or Mahayana teachings into the mainstream of Buddhist practice, sets forth the two opposing views succinctly in his *Treatise on the Middle Way*:

The Lower Schools:

> If all these are empty (of inherent existence),
> There will be no arising and disintegration;
> For you even the four noble truths
> Will become non-existent.

The Consequentialist:

> If all these are not empty (of inherent existence),
> There will be no arising and disintegration;
> For you even the four noble truths
> Will become non-existent.

So the reasoning: The subject, a house, inherently exists because it arises in dependence on causes and conditions, would be a valid argument from the lower school's point of view. A house inherently exists. The bricks and building materials that it is made of inherently exist and the atoms and so forth that make up the building materials also inherently exists. If the parts of the house were not inherently existent, they argue, when you put them together how would you have a house? For example, we may dream about building a house. We may dream that we have the various building materials. However, we obviously cannot build a real house with these dream materials. Why not? Because, as we discover when we awake, such materials were just in the nature of appearance, and not established from their own side. Compare the image of a person projected on to a screen by a film projector with a real person: with respect to these two different appearances of a person, on what basis, asks the proponents of the lower school's views, can the Consequentialist identify which is actually a person and which is not? For the lower schools it is easy. The projected image is not a person but is the mere appearance of a person, because from the side of the object there is not person to be found, as it were, to back up the appearance. The real person is a person because he is established from his own side as such. The Consequentialists' position is that nothing exists from its own side. Therefore they must accept the absurd consequence that, according to their view, there is no valid means to discriminate between the film image of a person and an actual person!

Moreover, if the state of liberation or enlightenment was not established from its own side but was just imputed by the mind, being some kind of mental projection, what reason would there be for attaining such a thing, and what benefit would there be in it? If the 'I' were merely mentally imputed how could we migrate from one life to the next? How could we experience pleasure and pain? If virtue and non-virtue, positive and negative actions were devoid of inherent existence what meaning would there be in engaging in one and abandoning the other? According to this critique by the lower schools then, the error of those who propound no inherent existence is so great that in their system the idea of such a thing as the path to liberation, the distinction between right and wrong and even the distinction between existence and non-existence lose all meaning.

In reply, the Consequentialists themselves admit that if one is a beginner in *dharma* practice, who doesn't have a very profound understanding of the teachings, then such an exposition as set forth by the lower schools, in which dependent-arising only refers to caused phenomena and is compatible with inherent existence, may well be a suitable basis for engaging in the *dharma*. Hearing that by practising virtue and abandoning non-virtue we can reach liberation can cause joy in some people and inspire them to take a new and wholesome direction in life. They feel great pleasure as if remembering something wonderful which they had always known but somehow had been temporarily forgotten or overlooked. Hearing nothing in this exposition by someone of the lower schools which contradicts their natural, instinctive assumption that all things inherent exist, then such a type of newcomer to the Buddha's teaching might feel all the more comfortable with their new outlook on life and thereby generate pleasure and enthusiasm in their practice.

The Buddha well understood that his ultimate teaching of no inherent existence would be beyond the range of some of his listeners' thought in the beginning and in view of this he taught the systems presented in the lower schools as lower steps or rungs by which such disciples might eventually reach an understanding of the highest explanation. But it would be mistaken to imagine that anyone can go either all the way to the enlightenment of a Buddha or to the lesser state of liberation from his or her own suffering in dependence on the lower school's view alone. To become free from cyclic existence it is indispensable that we meditate again and again on the ultimate mode of existence of phenomena, their emptiness of inherent existence. Being a subtle phenomena it is not easy to understand. We tend to have much more faith in the gross objects grasped by our senses. We have become very familiar over countless lifetimes with our way of seeing things as existing inherent, from their own side and we tend to cling to what we are familiar with. Nevertheless, by using the reasoning presented by the highest school of Buddhist thought, the Consequentialists, we will understand that this habitual mode of seeing is wrong and by persevering further we can wipe away the various layers of ignorance that encrust the natural purity of our mind.

IV

DEPENDENT-ARISING AND EMPTINESS: TWO VIEWS

The mind of crystal clarity that sees ultimate reality directly is developed through intensive meditation on the reasons which infallibly establish the nature of that reality. How dependent-arising is the chief of these reasons is the subject of this book. This is not to say that Buddhist path to freedom from suffering consists solely in training in reasoning and logic. The complete path has three divisions known as the three higher trainings, in moral discipline, concentration and wisdom. Then again, the type of Buddhism that spread and flourished in Tibet, Great Vehicle Buddhism, emphasizes the practice of compassion and concern for others to an extraordinary degree. However we have no space here to dwell on the teachings on moral discipline, concentration or compassion. Our subject falls into the category of wisdom which is not surprisingly where effort in reasoning is most needed. If we can develop the compassionate motivation to benefit all sentient beings impartially, that is excellent. In any case, if we can restrain our behaviour according to suitable moral guidelines, our mind will become steadier, less scattered and distracted. This gives us a suitable basis for building up a strong degree of concentration, which, when coupled with our wisdom-understanding will lead to insights. But before we can meditate productively on the ultimate nature of reality, which is indeed the meditation which will free us from the round of uncontrolled existence, we must first form a very clear picture of what it is and how to cultivate it. Arriving at even a clear mental image of it will for most of us require plenty of study, discussion, reflection and a willingness to try to reason things out. To try to proceed by intuition or meditation alone without bothering with these things may only lead to frustration, as in the following examples.

Suppose you have to tell a couple of children, possibly relatives of yours, to go to Moscow or some distant place, let us say to meet their father. Just letting them know that Moscow is in Russia, giving them a good reason for going there and telling them to go will not achieve a great deal. Being young children they have only the slightest idea of where Moscow and Russia are. Still less do they have any idea of how to get there, what documents they require and so forth. If they did set off on their own without any instructions, they would quickly get lost or become discouraged and give up, much as they might actually want to go. So what about someone who, hearing about nirvana or liberation and hearing that people reach nirvana by meditating on no-self and the emptiness of all phenomena, thereupon sits down with eyes closed, meditating with lots of inspiration and joyous enthusiasm...? Is not their quest equally certain to end in discouragement and failure? Or what if someone were given a gun and told to go out and shoot a deer, but that person had no idea what a deer looked like or where he was likely to find one. he might go out and fire his gun at something else. He might even shoot another person! The city of Moscow and the deer of our examples are far more easily recognizable objects than the subtler levels of ignorance that affect our minds. How much more carefully do we need to investigate and analyse therefore when trying to locate and eradicate our ignorance.

The practice of generosity and patience, refraining from harming others and developing compassion are greatly to be treasured. They must be practised by anyone who would imitate the Buddha or other great spiritual teachers, but the Consequentialist master Chandrakirti, highlighting the crucial importance of correctly identifying and vanquishing our root ignorance, call these good qualities 'eyeless.' In the *Supplement to the Middle Way*, he says:

> A single person with sight
> Can easily lead a group of blind people to their destination.
> Similarly a person who has the eyeless good qualities
> Can go to Buddhahood when guided by the wisdom seeing reality.

Looking more closely now at the views of the Buddhist schools below the Consequentialists, it is not so difficult to understand that caused phenomena or products are dependent-arisings in the sense that they arise in dependence on causes and conditions. A sprout comes forth from a seed. A child comes forth from his or her mother. The production of a sprout involves the coming together of an array of contributory factors. Soil or some similar medium is required in which there is the correct degree of moisture and warmth. If there is too much water the seed will rot; too little and will remain a seed. For its production it definitely relies on a host of things other than itself. But when we see a sprout once it has been produced, it appears to exist from its own side. it appears to possess its own intrinsic identity. So although it is not self-produced, it nevertheless appears to be self-reliant in the sense of possessing a nature that exists from within itself.

Very few people get round to questioning this appearance of inherent existence. The lower Buddhist schools assent to it. Whatever reservations some of them may have about other aspects of a sprout's mode of appearance, according to them all a sprout both appears to inherently exist and does so. The lower schools propound varying degrees of selflessness, some of great refinements, but none of them abandon the idea that the 'I' exists from its own side. Other objects appear to the self as if independent of it, not relying upon the 'I,' but existing in their own right. The lower schools assent to this and do not recognize that self and other depend on each other for their existence. They ask 'If objects did not have an identity independent of our observation of them, how could they act as a valid basis for our apprehension of them?'

According to them it is not in the basic way in which self and other are apprehended that is at fault; the problems begin when we develop exaggerated reactions to the self-existent 'I' and the self-existent other. We generate a neurotic attachment to the 'I' and cling to it and grasp at possessions, dear ones and allies, while developing impatience and exasperation for those who stand in our way, loathing for our enemies and envy for the possessions of rich and successful.

The fourth and highest school of Buddhist tenets, the Middle Way School, has, as we have said, two divisions, the Autonomists and the Consequentialists. The Autonomists, the lower of the two, put forward a further view of dependent-arising which is more extensive than that of the arising of effects in dependence on causes and embraces all phenomena. The explanation of dependent-arising furnished by the three lower schools is fine as far as it goes but it is incomplete, they say, because it fails to deal with permanent or uncaused phenomena.[6]

According to the Autonomists, if something is not a dependent-arising, then it does not exist. In the case of a table, not only does it depend on its causes, the wood from which it was made and so forth but it, the whole table, depends on its parts. When we perceive a table, the parts of a table, for example the legs, the smooth top, the parts nearer to the eye, the parts further away, the parts in the light and the parts in the shadow, apprehended together, go to make up the apprehension of a table. A person depend on his causes, his mother and father and so forth, and also he depends on his own parts or characteristics such as the colour of his skin, the shape of his body, his posture and habitual gestures, in the sense that only when someone apprehends sufficient of these features together are they able to apprehend him and discriminate him from anybody else.

Notice the shift in emphasis in this second explanation of dependent-arising away from the status of objects in their own right to a recognition of the interrelation of objects and subjects. This is a trend that we will find taken significantly further by the Consequentialists. The Autonomists still hold parts and whole to exist from their own side and to exist by way of

---

[6] Permanent phenomena are those phenomena which do not change and are not produced from causes. In this sense they are static, but not necessarily eternal. Existence itself is permanent. So are instance and generality, not any particular instance or generality but instance and generality themselves. True cessation (the third noble truth), which is the absence of all delusions in a realized being's mindstream, is another example, as is uncaused space, defined as the absence of obstruction and contact.

their own characteristics however. With respect to the mode of being of phenomena the Autonomists special position is that they assert a mode of being which is established from the object's own side, but which is posited through the power of appearing to a non-defective awareness. Their principal explanation of how phenomena are selfless therefore is that they are empty of existing from their own side without depending on being posited by a non-defective awareness. This is another way in which their view shows an advance in refinement over the lower schools. We may like to ask ourselves, for instance, whether the Autonomist views provides a better basis for explaining how different people see the same thing in slightly different ways.

From the highest point of view, that of the Consequentialists, the above explanation do not reveal the full import of reasoning of dependent-arising. Properly understood the reason of dependent-arising refutes any shadow of the existence of objects from their own side whatsoever. But it is very difficult to jump to the subtler explanations of dependent-arising straight away and one purpose of our introductory exploration of the other schools is to enable us first to focus precisely on just what the Consequentialists use the reasoning of dependent-arising to destroy–our instinctive assent to and grasping at the appearance of all and any phenomena to us as inherently existing, as having a mode of subsistence from the side of the object. If we think about and discuss the views of the other schools and then meditate on them and try to bring them within the realm of our own experience we will find that while some of the various assertions of the different schools contradict each other they all in the end contribute most helpfully towards shedding light on this instinctive, subtlest, most tenacious and most harmful ignorance of all.

A term which crops up frequently in debates between the schools about the precise nature of the ignorance that is the source of all the other delusions and just what antidote will eradicate it, is true existence. We have avoided using it much so far because it is one of those terms which different schools interpret in different ways, but thinking about it will give another slant to our understanding of what the Consequentialists single out as the key object of refutation. According to the Consequentialist interpretation, inherent existence, existence from the side of the object and true existence are all synonymous, so that for the Consequentialists nothing truly exists, which is by no means the same as saying that nothing is true and that everything is false, as we shall attempt to explain. We can approach the problem first by considering the term false. Three different usages of the term false can be distinguished. The first is the way the word is most commonly used in the world. If someone accuses us of stealing something when we have done nothing of the kind, then the statement of the other person is obviously false. Or our senses may be deceived, for instance when we are sitting in a stationary train but have the distinct impression that it is moving, only to realize a few second later that it is another train which we can see out of the window that is in fact moving and our train has not moved at all. We can say the consciousness we had for those few seconds was a false consciousness. The second meaning of false that we can distinguish concerns what is false according to someone's tenets or beliefs. Having studied a particular political, religious or scientific system and adopted it, one judges something to be false according to that framework, for instance, someone who is holder of Buddhist views would regard the opinion that the mind is a material phenomena as false. The third usage of the word false is the one closely connected with the Buddhist presentation of the ultimate nature of phenomena and occurs in the phrase, false existent. All phenomena appear to an ordinary consciousness to exist from their own side, but when investigated are found to have no such mode of existence whatsoever. For this reason, according to the Consequentialists, all phenomena are falsely existent and therefore non-truly existent. They are so not because they don't exist, but because they do not exist in the way they appear to our ordinary consciousness. In our first usage of the word false, some phenomena are false, such as the water of a mirage which is not water at all, and some are true, such as water, but all phenomena–even those which are true in the first sense–are false existent. So a holder of the Consequentialist point of view can assert that no phenomena truly or inherently exists but within that still discriminate between water that really is wet and water that is merely a mirage on a hot day. The Autonomists and Mind-Only followers have somewhat different notions of exactly what discrepancy between appearance and actuality the words non-truly existent should denote, but we will not venture into that here.

The phenomena depend on conditions is sufficient to establish for the Consequentialists, Tsongkhapa included, that they are empty of inherent existence. The lower schools disagree and hold completely the opposite view, that anything which depends on causes and conditions is necessarily inherently existent. We have sketched in the points of view of some of the lower schools and have tried to give the reasons why they think as they do. Ideally we should first try to see things in the way that the lower schools do. In that way their flaws, the areas in which their explanations leave us feeling dissatisfied, might become apparent to us. If we reach this point, then we will be in a position to readily absorb the Consequentialist view, and those who do directly understand that phenomena both arise in dependence upon conditions and are thereby empty of true existence are said to develop a sublime kind of joy and a profound faith in the teacher Buddha, since they thereby penetrate to the very essence of the teachings and generate the actual path to freedom. Those fortunate ones who gain this direct realization glorify Buddha and his teaching although few have done it as eloquently as Tsongkhapa.

The data we began with is again that all objects appear to have their own intrinsic identity residing within the object or from the side of the object. All objects appear to exist by way of their own intrinsic nature. Water's nature is to be wet with the power of moistening. Fire's nature is to be hot with the power of burning. But if water and fire had those characteristics from their own side then this means that they would not depend on any other phenomena for those characteristics. This would mean that any particular fire could never go out. If its hot and burning nature were independent of any other phenomena then what could act to extinguish it and how could it ever die out for lack of fuel? If a seed and a sprout were both established inherently, with their own intrinsic natures then the sprout would not arise in dependence on the seed and the seed would not produce it. Yet what meaning does the word seed have? A seed is something which has the capacity to produce a sprout. But if the entities of the seed and the sprout each existed from their own side, through their own power, then they would be unrelated. A seed's nature could not transform into the nature of a sprout. Another synonym for existence from the side of the object and inherently existent, according to the Consequentialists, is existence by way of the object's own characteristics. If we do not understand this term properly, like the term non-truly existent, it could lead us astray. We are not suggesting that a sprout and fire have no characteristics or nature of their own. What we mean is that these characteristics are not intrinsic to those objects, because then the fault would arise that since these characteristics would be independent of any affecting factors, the object would neither gain nor lose characteristics and could never transform into anything else or cease to exist.

When we set about meditating try to uproot our intrinsic grasping at inherent existence, the most important object to dwell on is the 'I.' If we consider how we ordinarily grasp at the 'I,' we tend to apprehend it as a very solid, independent phenomena that is able to set itself up from its own side. This is especially apparent if we observe the 'I' when we are in a state of strong emotion such as anger, fear, desire, or happiness. This is the best time to check up on the false mode of appearance of the 'I,' when we are strongly moved. But if the 'I' were really an independent object, then it could not be said to depend on the mind or body for its existence. So then, if we had a pain in our body, in our arm for example, there would be reason to say, 'I have a pain.' But if someone asked us, 'Are you experiencing pain?' then could we not correctly answer, 'yes,' and pointing to our arm say, 'I am experiencing pain in my arm?' Are these statements false, or do they reveal a dependent relationship between the 'I' and the body?

Surely the 'I' cannot be separated from and therefore depends on its parts, the mind and body. The mind is not the 'I' and the body is not the 'I.' The 'I' depends on for its identity on things which are not it, so the assertions of the lower schools that it has an intrinsic identity or that it exists inherently cannot be substantiated.

In another sense the 'I' is dependent because it depends on others. In order to distinguish the 'I,' we have to distinguish it *from others*. If we are to identify one object as self, we have, at the same time, to establish another category, other or others, for the term self to have any meaning. It is the same with the terms here and there. The place where we are now, we call here, but if there were no there to contrast it with how could the term be understood? Furthermore, to a person on the other side of the room, or road, or valley or whatever, from their point of view, where they are located is here and where we are is there. So for one particular place there are two different apprehensions, one valid for each of the two observers. Neither place is intrinsically here or there. The 'hereness' or 'thereness' is clearly not established from the side of object. Hot and cold, beautiful and ugly, pleasant and unpleasant and generality and particular are similar pairs of terms which are mutually dependent. None of the individual terms have an identity in their own right, or are able to set themselves up from their own side.

We have briefly mentioned three ways in which the 'I' or the 'self' is a dependent phenomena. It depends on its parts, it depends on others and it depends on the point of view of who is using the term. If we could devote time to any one of these modes of dependent-arising of the self and cause the strength of our habitual misapprehension of the self as autonomous and as established by way of its own characteristics to subside, at least to some extent, it would be very beneficial. We are not attempting to get rid of a sense of 'I,' only of the idea of this 'I' as self-existent or as established from its own side. Why should we try to get rid of the idea of the 'I' as self-existent and established from its own side? Because this is a false notion that obscures what is really the case and when we act on the basis of a misunderstanding we are likely to act unskillfully and end up causing problems for ourself and others. For instance, if we think we know a particular subject very well and develop pride in our knowledge, or even if we have a handsome and expensive house or car and we become proud about that and swagger about it, people are going to find it somewhat harder to like us. But then if we think more realistically about our level of knowledge or the quality of our house or car and compare ourselves not just with those people who are less well off than us in this or that respect, but also with the many who are far better off–much more knowledgeable, or possessing a really fabulous house or car–then our pride will decrease and people will find us less obnoxious, though of course our knowledge will not have decreased or will the value of our house or car have gone down. Similarly, thinking more realistically about how the self exists, in the way the Consequentialists propose, will not cause our sense of self to disappear but simply align it better with reality. This will bestow peace of mind, which is the object of the exercise.

The term conditions in the first line of the fifth verse, 'Whatever depends on causes and conditions,' is another term which is used differently by the lower schools and the Consequentialists. To the lower schools a condition is similar to a cause. Causes and conditions are what produce caused or impermanent phenomena such as consciousness, trees and mountains. The main object or objects which transform into a particular thing can be thought of as the cause of that result while the other contributory factors which may arise only just prior to the formation of the effect can be thought of as the conditions. For instance, in Tibetans medicine there is a category of illness which are of a hot nature and a category of those which are of a cold nature. When someone who has a complaint of a cold nature goes out in cold weather the illness manifests and they start to feel unwell. The illness itself is something which has a causal sequence beginning well before the present occasion. The cold weather is on the other hand the temporary condition which causes the symptoms to manifest strongly so that the person feels indisposed. The Consequentialists, however, also say that it is not only caused or impermanent phenomena that arise in dependence on conditions. The dependent relationship we mentioned earlier between here and there, generality and particular, beautiful and ugly, part and part-possessor and so forth are such that these phenomena are also said to arise in dependence upon conditions, without their necessarily being products or impermanent phenomena. Also all phenomena, both those which are produced and those which are not, have conception as one of the conditions for their establishment. For example, someone decides to make a vase for holding flowers in. First of all they hold a concept of the vase in their mind, that is they have a mental picture of the vase they want to create in their mind's eye. Then they actually go about to manufacture the vase. When it is finished, it is given the name, a vase. This name is applied to it by a conceptual mind to distinguish it from other objects. Take America as another example. Before westerners arrived there was obviously land there, but only after they arrived was the land named America, and not until the concept of America was formulated and the name America applied could anyone know what America was. All phenomena are designated by conception and so conception is one of the conditions of any phenomenon's establishment. Thus the Consequentialists hold that 'Whatever depends on conditions...' refers to all phenomena in that all phenomena are established in dependence on conditions. However, not all phenomena are *created* in dependence upon conditions. That only applies to impermanent phenomena.

In summary, when we apprehend an object such as a table, we apprehend an object that is produced in dependence on an infinite series of causes whose many different parts, the colour, the shape, the top, the sides, the legs and so forth, go to make up our apprehension of it, but the way a table appears to us, whether we look directly at one whether we close our eyes and think about one, is that it appears to have a nature which exists from its own side; this is a sense of 'tableness' appearing to reside right there within the object. When an object appears to set itself up like this, appearing not to depend on any other phenomena, the apprehension we have at that time is an apprehension of a truly existent, or an inherently existent object, that exists from its own side, by way of its own characteristics. Conversely, when we see a phenomena and clearly understand that the very existence of it is completely dependent on other phenomena, inseparably related to them, then at that time our mind is holding the view of dependent-arising. The basis for the apprehension of things as truly existent does not exist. There is no phenomena which exists independently of others. The basis for the apprehension of things as dependent-arising does exist. The only way phenomena do exist is an inter-dependently related. Obviously then, despite what the lower schools think, we cannot on the one hand accept inherent existence and also accept that phenomena inter-depend and, in the case of impermanent phenomena, cause each other. These two ways of existing are plainly contradictory.

5cd

What excellent instruction could there be
More amazing than these words?

...especially for someone who has followed the teachings of the lower schools and developed completely the opposite view! But for anybody, it is stressed, to realize the full import of dependent-arising, namely that all phenomena are empty of inherent existence, is an extremely forceful experience that reorients one in the very depths of one's being, cancels doubts and wrong views and bestows peace.

V

DEPENDENT-ARISING AND EMPTINESS: THE FINAL VIEW

6

Through wrongly holding (dependent-arising),
The childish strengthen bondage to extreme views.
But for the wise, the same thing is the means
To cut free from the net of elaborations.

In the first line of the sixth verse, those who wrongly hold or apprehend dependent-arising are all those who have not attained to the highest Consequentialist view of it and although all Buddhists would agree that Buddha taught a middle way, free from extremes, the highest Buddhist school, of which the Consequentialists are a sub-group, in particular characterize themselves as maintaining the true middle course, free from 'bondage to extreme views,' so much so that, as we may recall, they are named the Middle Way School. The extreme views are basically two. One is the abyss of nihilism. The unfortunates who plunge to this extreme are those who search through the aggregates of body and mind and like the Consequentialists come up with nothing substantial that they can point at and identify as the self. They then, unlike the Consequentialists, take it that the self does not exist and assume that the myriad objects of knowledge are also merely mistaken appearances, *maya* or illusion. Life for them becomes a meaningless game, devoid of any high purpose, with no distinction possible between good and bad or truth and falsehood, at best an exercise in keeping the upper lip stiff.

The other extreme is the abyss of permanence. Those who plunge to this extreme identify something either amongst the aggregates of body and mind or apart from them as an inherently existing 'I,' grasps strongly at a fixed essence to the person and possibly also at an unchanging essence in objects that endures throughout all the superficial changes in their outward semblance. Such a strong grasping at an inherently existent 'I' and 'mine' is the ideal basis for the poisonous delusions of desirous attachment and aversion to come springing forth. These delusions in turn motivate negative actions and thus the perpetuation of cyclic existence is assured. 'The wise,' on the other hand, use the reasoning of dependent-arising to steer away from the abysses of nihilism and permanence and arrive at the correct and liberating view of phenomena as empty of inherent existence. In another image, understanding dependent-arising will enable us to cut through the 'net of elaborations.' Elaborations are the countless misconceptions generated by the mistaken appearances of reality that all sentient beings have. The mistaken appearance above all is that of inherent existence of course and under its influence many paths, supposedly to complete happiness but merely leading up many cul-de-sacs to only limited partial happiness, have been explained. We have mentioned some of these alternatives above. There is the path of absolute inaction by which the practitioner thinks to attain liberation by exhausting all his or her previous *karma* without accumulating any fresh actions. There is the method of mental vacuity practised by those who see thought as the root of all problems and try to gain liberation by focussing the mind on nothingness in meditation. There are also in India practitioners who engage in various forms of physical endurance of pain, fasting and asceticism in the belief this will bring about an end to their negative *karma* and thus lead to freedom from suffering. Buddha himself spent six years in an experiment with asceticism before rejecting it as a path to liberation. Buddhism also stands apart from those religions the practice of which is largely devotional, validated by revealed truth alone, for we contend that final happiness comes about through understanding and that understanding can be achieved through application of reason. So also to those who picture the world as an endless maze with a middle course, or as a fundamentally random jumble of events, in other words to those who feel that the net of fabrications can never be ripped apart, we say, in the words of the Middle Way master Aryadeva in his treatise *The Four Hundred*,

> When dependent-arising is seen,
> Ignorance is not generated.
> Insight into selfless nature of phenomena
> Destroys the seed of cyclic existence.

In order to try to understand the subtlest explanation of the root ignorance, as delineated by the Consequentialists, we have sketched in the helpful, though incomplete, explanations of the lower schools concerning the mode of existence of phenomena in general. The lower schools also have their own special explanations of this root ignorance specifically in terms of the 'I' or 'self.' Ignorance concerning the 'I' is generally recognised as the most pernicious kind of ignorance because it is primarily due to misconceiving the nature of the 'I' that the disturbing attitudes of clinging attachment, jealousy, anger and pride come about. If we understand the Consequentialist point of view well, we shall see that there is, in fact, no difference between the kind of ignorance that obscures our view of the self and the kind of ignorance that obscures our view of other phenomena. In both cases it is the ignorance which superimposes the appearance of inherent existence on to the object. In the lower schools on the other hand distinctions are drawn between the ignorance regarding the elf and the ignorance regarding other phenomena, so two different kinds of ignorance are described in each of these schools. Here we will merely pick out the two main misconceptions of the 'I' that the lower schools say must be eradicated in order to gain liberation and contrast them with what the Consequentialists say is the root ignorance that binds us to the wheel of existence.

The first wrong conception of the 'I' that the lower schools refute is the apprehension of the 'I' as permanent, single and independent. This is an 'I' which is permanent because it is without production and disintegration, single in the sense that is it without parts and independent because it does not depend on the aggregates or anything else. It is like a pea in a jar, the jar being the aggregates of body and mind and the pea being the 'I' residing within the aggregates until the aggregates disintegrate at death, at which point the 'I' goes on to its next rebirth. The second misconception of the 'I' is grasping the 'I' to be the substantially established in the sense of being self sufficient. This misapprehension is subtler than the former and is held to be the main obstacle to individual liberation by the schools below the Consequentialists. It is the conception of the existence of a self which is capable of being identified independently, without relying on the identification of the aggregates. The feeling one has when grasping at this 'I' is of there being something to which all the aggregates belong, and owner or governor of them, something which has a different character to them and possesses them, thinking 'mine.'

According to the Consequentialists, while it is necessary to abandon these two levels of ignorance, that alone is not sufficient to cut free of the net of elaborations concerning the self. To do that we need to abandon not just these two gross levels of self-grasping but also the subtler level of grasping at the self to be inherently existent. To refute the first false notion of the 'I' we would do well to consider why the 'I' must be impermanent. Our bodies and our minds are changing from moment to moment. Both a person and the parts of that person are effects and at the same time causes involved in a continual process of transformation. Is there any place for a permanent, i.e., unchanging 'I' or 'self' in all this? With regard to the second false apprehension of 'I' we have to break down our instinctive grasping at an independently identifiable 'I,' controlling the aggregates, but not relying on them. To counter this attitude we have to investigate how the apprehension of the self always depends on apprehending some other phenomena. We recognize somebody only by apprehending some part of them, their face or general shape, perhaps. If it is somebody we know very well we can recognize them just be hearing their cough or the sound of their footstep. However the self exists, it does not exist over and above the aggregates but is inseparable from them. The subtlest self grasping, grasping the self to be inherently existent, is countered by applying arguments to establish that a self existing either from the side of the aggregates or separate from them is completely unfindable. We have to mentally search again and again through the parts of the self, all through the body and the mind, to convince ourselves no one part is the self, anymore than we can isolate one part of a telephone from the rest of the parts and say "That is the telephone." Our body is not the self. If it was, how could we say, "I am thinking?" Our mental consciousness is not the self. Otherwise how could we say, "Somebody touched me" or "I kicked the ball?" Although it is completely contrary to the way we normally apprehend ourselves, reasoning shows that among the parts of the mind and body there is nothing that we can point to and say, "This is the 'I'." We should extend the search for the 'I' outside the aggregates to convince ourselves that there is no 'I' which exists completely separate from its part either. The next stage is to familiarize ourselves deeply with the absence of an 'I' that exists by way of its own entity, by going over this reasoning again and again, and gradually our habitual self-grasping will lose its power.[7]

Finally, one telling difference between the lower schools and the Consequentialists is that the former all agree that, after removing the superimpositions or false appearances of the self, the actual 'I' can be identified within the aggregates and, as it were, pointed out. To take one example, the Autonomists, the other followers of the Middle Way School, apart from the Consequentialists, point to some form of the mental consciousness as the 'I.' The Consequentialists, on the other hand, refute any suggestion that the actual 'I' can be found within the aggregates and only speak of an 'I' which is designated to its basis of designation, the parts of the 'I,' by the conceptual mind.

---

[7] For further details on how to conduct a basic meditation on the absence of inherent existence of the 'I,' see the early sections of *Meditation on Emptiness* by Jeffrey Hopkins.

7

Since this teaching is not found elsewhere,
You alone are the 'Teacher.'
For a Tirthika, this name would be a flattery,
Like calling a fox a lion.

8

O wondrous teacher! O wondrous refuge!
Supreme speaker! Great Protector!
I pay homage to the Great Teacher
Who so clearly explained dependent-arising.

In the first line of seventh verse 'teaching' refers to the teaching of emptiness of inherent existence of all phenomena by the reason of dependent-arising. 'This teaching is not found elsewhere' asserts that it is unique to the Buddhist canon. Furthermore, it is only distinguished in the commentaries of Consequentialists, being overlooked by the philosophers even of the other Buddhist schools. 'Tirthika' was the Sanskrit term employed by Buddhist writers for the followers of other non-Buddhist Indian philosophical schools. One way of explaining the four epithets for the Buddha in the eighth verse is to say that 'wondrous teacher' refers to the Buddha as the teacher of the lower schools tenets, where he did not deny inherent existence, and 'wondrous refuge' is a praise to the Buddha for teaching the highest system of tenets in which the inseparability of emptiness and dependent-arising is revealed. Understanding this is our ultimate refuge from the suffering of cyclic existence. 'Supreme speaker' refers to the Buddha's teaching of the lower schools' view again, in accordance with the needs of those of lesser capacity and 'Great Protector' is again a description merited by the Buddha's ultimate teaching on dependent-arising and emptiness for the students of great capacity. This verse, the eighth, is called the homage of the main text whereas the first verse was the homage of the introduction.

9

O Benefactor! To heal all beings
You proclaimed (dependent-arising),
The peerless reason for ascertaining
Emptiness, the heart of the teaching.

10

How could those who see
The way of profound dependent-arising
As contradictory or unproven
Ever understand your system?

That which destroys cyclic existence from the root is the meditation on the emptiness of inherent existence of the self and phenomena. Dependent-arising is the peerless reasoning to understand it. Sometimes dependent-arising is called, 'king of reasonings.' The non-Buddhist philosophical schools, for example the Hindu schools of India, are the ones who, when presented with a reasoning such as: 'Considering the subject, the self; it is empty of inherent existence because it is a dependent-arising,' would be most likely to reply that the reason in the above syllogism, 'because it is a dependent-arising' was not proven. The lower Buddhist schools are the ones who would most probably answer by saying that the reason was contradictory, since for them something's being a dependent-arising is a sign that it is inherent existent. We mentioned some of the lower schools counter arguments in chapter III, using the examples of the film image of a man and a house seen in a dream. We can now try to answer these objections, though first we will restate them with a couple of more illustrations. The first is when someone sees a length of rope in the grass at dusk and panics, thinking he or she is about to tread on a snake. Clearly the thing lurking in the grass from its own side is not a snake. There is merely somebody imputing a snake in that place. Consequentialists have to admit that a real snake is very similar to the imaginary snake in this situation because they hold the real snake also to be merely imputed, lacking an identity as a snake from the side of the object. Therefore does not the Consequentialist have to accept the absurdity that, according to his own tenets, the imaginary snake is a real snake since he has no valid means to discriminate between them? Compare dream experiences with experiences of the waking state: since both sets of experiences are merely projected by the mind and have no true existence, no distinction can be drawn between them in terms of whether the experiences are actual or not. If, for example, a fully ordained monk (who has strict vows against killing) dreamed that he deliberately murdered someone and rejoiced in having done so, would not he have broken his vows? In his dream he only killed a person who was merely imputed, but so what? The Consequentialists would have you believe that even a person whom you might kill during the waking state has no mode of existence other than a mere imputation by conception.

In fact these questions were posed quite some time ago. The question about killing in a dream is recorded in sutra as having been asked of the Buddha himself, while the question about the rope and the snake was dealt with by Nagarjuna, the great Indian commentator. Unfortunately this does not mean that it is possible to formulate the answers very simply. When the lower school debaters hear the Consequentialists say that all phenomena are merely imputations, they assume that this signifies that all phenomena are merely imaginary. They say that to call something a mere imputation denies the existence of any object at all except for some conjured up figment of the imagination. The Consequentialists are only denying that objects exist by way of their own characteristics which of course to them is very different from denying objects altogether. So Consequentialists say in reply that when we impute an object it is certainly necessary to have a valid basis for such an imputation. A rope for instance is not a valid basis on which to impute a snake.

The lower schools, on their part, say that a piece of rope is not a snake simply because it is not a snake from its own side, and that a real snake is a snake because it is a snake from its own side. This explanation fails to acknowledge the exclusive role of imputation in conceiving and identifying objects. In order to demonstrate how a phenomenon can be *merely* imputed by the mind apprehending it, consider the following example: suppose somebody produces a superb forgery of a hundred rupee note, so good that only the most experienced experts at the national mint can tell the difference between it and the real thing. In quality of paper, engraving and colouring the fake is virtually identical with an actual one hundred rupee note; only one or two minute details distinguish it. Of these virtually identical scraps of paper, how does one come to be worth one hundred rupees, while the other fit only to be shredded? It is simply because the experts, with the backing of the legal system, pronounce one to be real money, having that face value and pronounce the other to be worthless. Purely through the force of imputation then, one piece of paper is exchangeable for a hundred rupees worth of goods while the other has no value. In the case of a snake, someone at a certain time in the past first gave the name snake to a certain object, the animal with the characteristics unique to snakes. To the basis they applied the designation 'snake.' Just so today, when enough of those characteristics, the sinuous body, the absence of legs, the patterned skin, the fangs and so on, appear to mind, we may validly impute snake to that set of characteristics. In our example of a length of a rope lying on the ground in the twilight, on the basis of an appearance to mind of a sinuous, legless animal with poison fangs lurking in the grass, the person walking in the dusk apprehends snake and recoils in horror. But if he takes a close look at the object in the grass, although he will see a sinuous legless form, he will see nothing he could call a body or a possessor of fangs, nothing he could call a head or tail, nothing he could call an animal even. So a closer examination of the basis of imputation, the rope, reveals that it is not something to which one can ascribe the uncommon characteristics of a snake and therefore it is unsuitable to apprehend it as a snake. There are two significant differences between the mind which apprehends an actual snake and one that apprehends a rope as a snake. Firstly we cannot ascribe to the rope the qualities of having a body or fangs or a forked tongue or the qualities of being able to crawl on its belly along the ground or to bite other creatures. Therefore it is not a fit basis for the designation snake. Secondly, if the person who originally thought the rope was a snake takes a second, closer, look then he will be able to see that the rope is not a snake but a rope. This latter perception, of a rope lying in the grass, is a correct or valid perception and it establishes that the former perception, of the rope as a snake, was mistaken. It is capable of overturning the former perception; in other words the former perception can be disproven. Therefore a rope is not a basis for the designation, snake.

If we are asked whether the object designated, the snake, resides within the basis of designation, the characteristics or parts, we have to answer that indeed it does not. For instance, the skin of the snake is not the snake; the long thin body is not the snake; nor are the fangs, nor any of the other features either individually or collectively. The fact is that a conceptual mind apprehends a snake by imputing it on to a number of characteristics which appear to that mind, none of which are themselves a snake. People who say that a snake exists by way of its own entity or from its own side are obliged to come up with something among the parts, features or characteristics of a snake that it essentially the snake. Unless they are able to put forward something substantial like that to point at as the actual object or at least a substantial basis on which to hand their imputation, they have to acknowledge that the snake is merely imputed. In the case of sentient beings, most of the lower schools posit the mental consciousness in one form or another as this substantial factor which is the inherent essence of that being. In the case of inanimate objects it is somewhat harder to point to any individual features as the essence of the object. The two lowest schools, The Particularists and the Sutra-followers, say at this point that, in the case of inanimate objects, the collection the parts of the object is the object. For instance, the collection of the parts of a motor car is a motor car. To this the Consequentialists respond, "If all the parts of a car were dumped anyhow in a heap in front of you, the collection of parts would be there but they would not cause you to think 'That is a car.' Therefore it is incorrect to say that the collection of the parts of a car is a car." The followers of Mind Only and the Autonomists on their part put forward the distinctive shape or arrangement of the parts of the object as the object. To them the Consequentialists respond, "Where is this distinctive shape or arrangement of parts of the car? No individual part possesses it. Instead of existing from the side of the parts, is not this distinctive shape or arrangement of parts something designated to them when they are assembled?" This is contrary with the car's supposed findability or ability to be located within the object. Thus this shape or arrangement of parts does not fulfill the criterion of being something which, from its own side, is the car.

Consider the person who made the first car. First he had a concept of what he wanted to invent. Then he set about making it. After a few prototypes perhaps, he finally made something which fulfilled his concept. It was able to perform the function of the object he had in mind in the way intended. At this point he designated what he had made as car. All the other cars that have come into the world since then are apprehended in the same way. On the basis of an appearance to mind of the assembled components that are able to perform that particular function the mind imputes, car. What can we say of ultimate nature of a car other than that it is devoid of any existence from its own side, in the first place because it depends on causes and conditions, in the second place because it depends on its parts and in the third place because it depends on the three, a base of designation, a conceptual mind which designates it and a term to designate it by?

The second problem posed by the advocates of lower school views who are looking for weaknesses in the Consequentialist position concerns the monk who kills someone in a dream. All the schools can agree that the dream victim is not real person because he does not possess the defining characteristics of a person From the lower schools point of view he does not possess the defining characteristics of a person first and foremost because he is not a person who exists from his own side; this is because he is merely an appearance in somebody's dream. From the Consequentialists' point of view real people do not exist from their own side any more than the ones who appear in dreams. But from their perspective the dream victim does not possess the defining characteristics of a person because, however real he appears to the dreamer during the short time of the dream state, he is not someone who has the ability to speak, to think for himself, to accumulate *karma* and so on. A real person has to have a certain history too. A real person is born at a certain time in a certain place. It is to some such variety of characteristics as these, embodied only by a person, that the term person or human is suitable to be applied. If the term human or person is applied to any other base of designation such as a figment of imagination in a dream, the film image of a person or the reflection of a person in a mirror then the term is being used incorrectly. From the point of view of their not existing from their own side the real person and the dream person are the same. From the point of view of the way ordinary objects are understood and the way terminology is conventionally used, there is all the difference in the world.

Thus the monk in the example does not accumulate the negative action of killing a person. It is said that some negative *karma* of a lesser kind may be accumulated due to the generation of the intention to kill in a dream. Generally dreams are a reflection of the actions, mental or physical that one has engaged in during the waking state. Imprints from these actions can manifest during the time of sleep. If one has engaged in very negative actions this can be reflected in nightmares, while it is said that if one has performed many virtuous actions one will have pleasant dreams. There is another type of dream, which is much less common, when the mind becomes very clear and events that are yet to occur are revealed to us. Sometimes also in a dream we can receive an indication or confirmation that a spirit or evil influence is trying to harm us. There might be other occasions when, if one has a particular strong affinity with one's own meditational deity, this deity can reveal certain things and bestow blessings during a dream. There is also a yogic practice where the adept can use the mind which manifests at the time of sleep. One characteristic of the mind of sleep is that it is, like the mind at the point of death, subtler than the ordinary gross waking consciousness. If one uses this level of consciousness to meditate on certain objects, this can bring about realisations. Here we are talking about somebody with a highly developed mind. Apart from these special cases the majority of dreams are said to arise from the awakening of the latent impressions left by the actions we are most familiar with.

VI

IN DAILY LIFE

11

When one perceives 'empty'
As the meaning of 'dependent-arising,'
Empty of inherent existence does not contradict
The function of agent and action.

12

Whereas if one perceives the opposite,
Since there can be neither action in emptiness
Nor emptiness in what has action,
One would fall into a dreadful abyss.

13

Therefore, understanding dependent-arising,
As you have taught, is well praised.
(Things) are not totally non-existent,
Nor are they inherently existent.

14

The independent is like a sky-flower,
Therefore nothing is not dependent.
Existence with self-nature precludes
Establishment by causes and conditions.

Others see the reasoning of dependent-arising as unproven, or contradictory with that which it is designed to prove, namely that all phenomena are empty of inherent existence. Tsongkhapa relied on the interpretations of the Consequentialist school and realised that emptiness and dependent-arising are supremely harmonious. With this realisation, all his perplexities concerning the ultimate import of Buddha's teaching were dissolved. Perceiving that emptiness of inherent existence and dependent-arising are completely compatible is the incomparable insight of those who actualize the Buddha's highest teachings and is the deepest well-spring of their faith. We can deepen and extend our appreciation of the various facets of dependent-arising by considering it under three headings, depending, relying and meeting or connecting. Even if we feel we are a long way from achieving Tsongkhapa's level of illumination and insight, contemplating these different aspects of dependent-arising is a sure way to develop our good qualities of generosity, tolerance and concern for others.

The first of the three aspects, depending, embraces the simplest level of dependent-arising, that of effects being the product of causes. Considering how effects are dependent on causes is in itself a great antidote to self-centered and self-satisfied attitudes which lead to our being insensitive to the predicament of others and dismissive of the complexity of their problems. When we are doing fine we do not notice how the kindness of many other beings has contributed to our happiness. When we are down we lunge for a simplest explanation which places all the blame on others. For instance we probably all have the tendency to think that whatever good health we have to a large extent comes about through our own vigilance and whatever experiences we enjoy are the deserved fruits of our own hard work. Our analysis of how the good conditions we enjoy arise often tends to go no further than some such though as "I know how to take care of myself,' or 'I put in a lot of effort to be able to afford this." If we go to a restaurant and have a delicious meal, superficially we might think that being able to do this just depends on our own means, having earned enough money to pay for it. However, if we investigate exactly what being able to eat a meal in a restaurant really depends on, we will see that in fact an enormous amount of effort has to be put in by countless number of beings before we can be served our choice of food. If we are eating rice, we can think of all the work of the farmers, ploughing, planting, weeding, irrigating and finally harvesting their crops. Of course all the labour of themselves and their draught animals would be in vain if the elements did not cooperate and provide the right amount of sunshine and rain. Then the rice has to be cleaned and milled and prepare for the table. Then it is distributed and put on sale in the shops. Another network of people is required. Once the rice has reached the restaurant, the kitchen staff have to work hard on the final stage of the process of making it fit to eat. The kitchen and the dining room themselves are the fruits of the labour of gangs of people and the cook's utensils, the fuel for cooking and the serving dishes have only come into being in dependence on the inventiveness, ingenuity and effort of another vast number of designers, administrators, sales people, accountants, factory worker, miners and then all their families and teachers and so forth.

In Mcleod Ganj, where His Holiness the Dalai lama lives, there are a considerable number of restaurants catering largely to the westerners and other visitors who come on pilgrimage, to study or just as tourists. As the number of the visitors has increased so have the hotel and restaurant facilities expanded. Clearly the visitors depend on the restaurants and hotels and equally the hotel and restaurant workers depend on the visitors. As the range of facilities for visitors improves, so are more people tempted to come, and as the number of visitors increases, so do more people take to the business of selling them food, souvenirs, handicrafts and books on Buddhism. Many of the Tibetan shop and hotel owners would say that this situation ultimately rests on the kindness of His Holiness and the Three Jewels.[8] They are very happy to see the visitors from other parts of India and the rest of the world who come to Mcleod Ganj, happy on their own account and also when they think of the benefit the visitors can derive from finding out about Buddhism. The visitors are pleased that facilities in McLeod Ganj are not so bad, and that they can get decent food there. They can appreciate the welcome they get and the cheerfulness of the Tibetans and they too can understand that there is mutual benefit for themselves and the Tibetans in their being there. But if either side were to lapse into a more self-centred way of thinking, such as "I am the one who built up this restaurant by my own hard work," or "I can eat at this expensive restaurant because I worked hard and saved up a lot of money," then, thinking that their fortunate situation did not depend on others, only on themselves, there would be a degeneration of this happy feeling between the two sides and the mutual tolerance of each others' foibles.

---

[8] The Three Jewels are the three objects a Buddhist goes to for refuge. They are the Buddha or Enlightened One, the Dharma, his teaching and the Sangha, the community of those who have made progress on the path to enlightenment.

Another example of the benefits of remembering dependent-arising occurs in the following story about a man who was going to market with a yak. As he was leading the yak along a mountain path the yak slipped and fell off the track. It fell into a narrow place in such a way that it was unable to rise again. So the man made a very strong prayer to the Buddhas, and to Padmasambhava in particular, and by heaving on the rope he was able to get the yak back on its feet. But instead of thinking about the kindness of the Buddhas or the Three Jewels, he set off again on his journey with a very inflated view of his own strength. A little further on the yak fell down again. This time the man thought he could get the yak back to its feet just by tugging on the rope, without bothering with the prayer, but try as he might the yak remained stuck and he could not shift it an inch! Whatever we undertake, if we remember that our success depends on far more than just our own prowess or wealth we will only be more in touch with the reality of the situation, since the dependent relationships of one phenomena with others are in fact countless. Being more in touch with the reality of our situation can only help us–in getting on better with other people for instance. As for the power of prayer, Padmasambhava was one of the first and greatest yogis to spread Buddha's teachings in Tibet and a prayer backed up by strong faith in him can help good *karma* to ripen at a certain point to bring about a desired result. Just as a child's willingness to learn makes it possible for the teacher to draw out the child's understanding, so, as in the story, making a prayer can help to draw out our ability to solve a particular problem at a critical time.

The second aspect of dependent-arising, relying, does not exclude the relationship between effects and causes we have discussed under the heading dependent, but also stressed in an explanation of relying is the mutual relationship between parts and wholes. We cannot have an apprehension of a table unless we apprehend some of the parts of a table and we cannot understand what a part of a table, such as a table leg or the colour of a table, is without understanding a table. If we are standing outside at night and we see a pair of lights flickering in the distance and then we hear the roar of a motor, we think, "There is a car coming." Simultaneous with the apprehension of a car is the understanding that the lights are the lights of a car and that the engine noise is the noise of a car. A car and the parts of a car, in this instance, its lights and its sound, rely upon each other. Neither is apprehended without the car. Another dimension of the concept of relying is the way in which pairs of things like self and other, short and tall, here and there and subject and object are mutually reliant. The only way self, for instance, can be distinguished is by contrasting it with other. If everyone were exactly the same size there would be no perceptions of small and tall people. To get a grasp of what a tall person is we must have some notion what a person who is not tall is like. Furthermore, a western man who comes to McLeod Ganj may find that Tibetans who see him think of him as tall or big on the basis that he is somewhat taller and more heavily built than most Tibetans. Back in his own country however he may be no more than average-sized person, who nobody thinks of as tall. It is only in reliance upon the appearance of other phenomena, and in comparison with them, that any particular object can be designated as big or small, beautiful or ugly, good or bad and so forth. If we are asked, "Is this big?" strictly speaking we cannot reply

'Big in relation to what?' Often the kind of perception we have of an object relies very much on past experience. Take momos for instance. Tibetans are very fond of these steamed dumplings especially when they are filled with meat. On the other hand, vegetarians or somebody who ate momos before and got very sick would perhaps find them most unpleasant to eat. In themselves are momos pleasant tasting, unpleasant, or neither? No general answer can be given, only an answer from a particular pint of view, in reliance upon a comparison with other tastes and flavours.

Meeting, the third aspect of dependent-arising explained by the Consequentialists, stresses the way in which a multitude of different factors come together in any act of cognition. For any object to be cognized there has to be the meeting of the object with the consciousness apprehending it. More specifically it is the parts of the object assembled together which cast their aspect to the mind and produce an apprehension of the object. Any entity we grasp at as having a single identity in fact results from many different aspects meeting or coming together to form it. As an example, take a product such as a knife. It comes about through the meeting of its causes, some iron for the blade and a piece of wood for the handle, the craftsmen involved the heat of the forge, the hammer and the cutting, grinding and polishing tolls. Then there is the coming together of its parts, the blade, the haft and rivets or glue which fasten them together. Finally the collection of parts meets with a consciousness which knows what the distinguishing characteristics of a knife are and that consciousness interprets the assemblage of parts as a knife.

Contemplating dependent-arising under the three headings of dependent-arising, relying and meeting will enrich our understanding and put at our fingertips many ways of reasoning against our ingrained grasping at inherent existence. When we recollect how thoroughly dependent our own existence is on the labour of multitude of other, will not that help to reduce our self-satisfied pride? When we consider that the people who are the object of our anger are not a worthy object of anger from their own side, but are merely grasped as such by our own rampaging mind, will not that rob our anger of the fuel that feeds it? Practically speaking, long before we are able to convince ourselves with watertight logical proof that all phenomena are utterly devoid of existence by their own power, we can use our limited understanding of dependent-arising to catch our negative emotions before they boil up and become really poisonous. Once we are in the throes of a fit of jealousy or rage our mind is generally too turbulent to steer onto a different course. But by analysing what went wrong afterwards and recollecting frequently the various facets of dependent-arising we can gradually reduce the frequency and intensity of our negative emotions.

Other benefits of remembering dependent-arising were spoken of by Buddha as three. Firstly, remembering dependent-arising will keep us from falling to either of the two extremes, the extreme of permanence or the extreme of nihilism. When we recollect that all things are interdependent, we will not grasp at ourselves and other phenomena as being inherently existent. By focusing on how all things are dependently-related we will realize that they can only be related in the first place by virtue of the fact that they exist. The first recognition will prevent us falling to the extreme of permanence and the second will prevent us from falling to the extreme of nihilism. Secondly, understanding dependent-arising will enable us to recognize correctly how phenomena exist only nominally through the conventions of terminology.The third benefit is that we will be able to understand clearly how phenomena are like a magician's illusions or reflections in water. Up until the verses quoted at the beginning of this chapter, the explanation of dependent-arising has been directed towards realizing the emptiness of inherent existence of phenomena. What the verses at the beginning of this section reveal is that understanding emptiness thoroughly leads one to a still better understanding of dependent-arising. The most profound aspects of dependent-arising, it is said, do not become clear until after one has realized emptiness.

We will come to Tsongkhapa's description of phenomena as being like illusions in a later verse, but the question of what this nominal existence is that is left after we have proved that phenomena do not exist by way of their own entities or characteristics is a pertinent one and is a point over which the Consequentialists part company with the other Buddhist schools. The other schools' position is that if one rejects inherent existence then it is tantamount to rejecting existence as such. Without inherent existence nothing would exist, or else any appearance to mind would have to be accepted as valid. The Consequentialists reply that just because what exists is merely imputed, it does not follow that whatever is imputed exists. A man who sees a rabbit in the distance with its ears sticking up might think that he is seeing a rabbit with horns. This does not mean that a horned rabbit exits. When the man thinks, 'That rabbit has got horns,' the basis of designation, an ordinary rabbit, and the object designated, a rabbit having horns, do not have the compatibility necessary for the imputation to stick, as we discussed earlier in our example of the rope and the snake. By abandoning the idea of there being a solid core, existing from the object's own side, on which the object can be designated, we can follow the Consequentialists' inspiration and experiment with the experience of all things as empty or selfless, but, unless we have a sound way to posit the things of the world such as cows, trees, chairs and rabbits we will only have succeeded in plunging to the abyss of nihilism. Two lines of thought which are exclusive to the Consequentialists can be set forth to indicate ways in which the existence of the phenomena of the world can be upheld after inherent existence has been repudiate. The first concerns the mutual reliance of parts and whole; the second concerns accepting things as merely nominally existent, dependent on terms or designates.

If we think about a sprout and ask where it came from we can say it came from a seed. The seed in turn was produced by an earlier plant, which itself was once a seed. The beginning of this process of seeds and sprouts producing each other is lost in time. The 'I' or 'self' is something which is apprehended in dependence on the aggregates or parts of a person. And what does the apprehension of a part such as the body depend on? It parts, the limbs, the torso and the head? Is the torso also only apprehended in dependence on its parts in turn, and those parts on their parts? Is the process of apprehending a person a virtually endless one when we examine it, like the process of the production of seeds and plants? This is surely rather an unwieldy way of positing the conventional person. Nevertheless, the lower schools are obliged to resort to this description of the process. They do not say the person is devoid of inherent existence of course. But, since they deny the existence of a person who is substantially existent in the sense of being self-sufficient, they have to be able to describe how a person can be imputed on to any of his or her aggregates. The Consequentialists, rather than going through this endless explanation simply say that a person is established in dependence on the aggregates of a person and the aggregates of a person are established in dependence upon a person.

For instance, suppose we are standing at the edge of a jungle and we hear the roar of an animal which we recognize to be the sound of a tiger. We can only recognize the sound as the sound of a tiger if we know what a tiger is and judge that there is no lurking in the undergrowth. At the same time, it is only the roar of the tiger that indicates to us the presence of a tiger, supposing we can neither see nor smell the beast. In this situation our realization of a tiger and the sound of tiger are simultaneous and mutually dependent. This is how those refute inherent existence affirm all the phenomena of the world, through their dependent relationships with each other. There is no fixed independent essence to any phenomena but phenomena are not thereby merely figments of our imagination like the child of a barren woman. When phenomena are imputed to their parts no endless chains of imputation of parts upon smaller parts are observed but the cognition of the whole and the parts each rely on the other. This reliance is like an old man who gets up with the aid of stick. In order to rise, the man leans on his stick. The man is therefore supported by his stick, but at the same time, the stick is supported by the man. Without the man to place the stick in the upright position and hold it, the stick would be unable to perform the function of bearing the man's weight. All phenomena participate in these relationships of mutual dependence. However, it is said that this aspect of dependent-arising only become completely clear after we have realized emptiness.

Understanding how to accept all things are mere designations means recognizing how they exist only nominally, through the conventions of terminology, which was classed above as the second benefit of realizing dependent-arising. As our example here we can take anger. Under the influence of anger our powers of sensible decision fly out of the window and we do many regrettable things. It is thus very beneficial, to control it. Discovering the emptiness of inherent existence of anger, the person who is angry and the object of anger is a supreme antidote but trying to apply this antidote once the anger has erupted is not easy. After the anger has subsided we should analyse it and try to isolate it. Anger manifests in various ways: we clench our muscles; our hearts beat faster; our face goes red; our voice rises to a scream; perhaps we pour forth stream of invective; we have a rampant blind urge to destroy the object of our anger, but we cannot point a finger at any of these manifestations and identify any one of them as the actual anger. Within the mind itself during the time we are angry, different aspects can be mentally identified: there is the feeling of being let down or deprived of something; there is also a feeling of grievance where the blame is focused on another person or an object; there is the part of the mind which instigates the action of lashing out with hand or tongue. None of these can be pinpointed as the actual anger. Analysing thoroughly in this fashion we arrive again at the point where we cannot find anything from the side of the object which is that object. We have a group of characteristics, none of which itself is anger, which between them amount to something which performs the function of anger. Anger is merely designated to this base of designation. If we perform an ultimate analysis, looking for the anger that exists from its own side, we find nothing. This mere absence constitutes the emptiness of inherent existence of anger and should be meditated on as much as possible. The only anger that can be found is one that exists merely in terms of a designation. One has to be satisfied with this mere nominal existence of anger simply because no other mode of existence can be identified.There are certain characteristics or manifestations which act as the basis of the designation. There is the consciousness which does the designating. Then there is the designation or term applied by that consciousness to that basis, according to the conventions of terminology. If we try to find something deeper, something underneath the name that is the object, we will be unsuccessful. We can only keep coming back to the designation itself. Again this is the subtle aspect of dependent-arising which the realization of emptiness is said to assist us in cognizing. So, dependent-arising is in the first place the supreme reasoning that leads to a realization of emptiness but then a realization of emptiness in turn leads back to a more thorough-going appreciation of dependent-arising.

If we thoroughly understand that anger and the person who is angry are empty of inherent existence, we will become free of our bondage to anger. But realising that things are not inherently existent should not lead us to reject conventional reality and view all discrimination as a hindrance. As the great Indian master of logic Dharmakirti says in his Commentary on Valid Cognition:

> With the aid of sounds, terms are imputed;
> This is for conventional (understanding).
> The purpose of words ends there -
> Is this clear to you?
>
> The skilful accept worldly conventions
> Because in dependence on them
> They can lead people to their object of attainment,
> The ultimate goal.

Verse 11 of Tsongkhapa's text indicates how closely emptiness of inherent existence and dependent-arising are related; one is the 'meaning' of the other, and the denial of inherent existence does not negate the phenomena of the world. Verse 12 indicates that those who cannot see that emptiness and dependent-arising are dependently related are making a fatal error. Either they cling to the reality of actions and reject emptiness, or they embrace emptiness and see all activity and discrimination as meaningless. In either case they tumble from the middle way into the abyss of perplexity. Most people's instinctive tendency is to go to the first extreme of grasping things to be inherently existent. They have to refute the inherent or 'independent' existence of things, which is like a sky flower or the horn of a rabbit, utterly non-existent. When one breaks down one's habitual assumptions and one first realizes that things are devoid of independent existence, at that time there is said to be a particular tendency to veer towards the other extreme of thinking that things are 'totally non-existent.'

VII

ILLUSION AND REALITY

15

Thus it is taught that because nothing exists
Other than the dependently-arisen
There is no existing thing
Which is not empty of inherent existence.

16

Since inherent nature has no end, you said that
Nirvana would be impossible
If phenomena had any inherent nature,
For elaborations could not be stopped.

Verse 15 and 16 develop the main theme of the *Praise for Dependent-Arising*; that there is no phenomena of the past, present or future that is inherently existent and not dependently existent. Being inherently existent is simply impossible. If something was inherently or intrinsically established then no causes or circumstances could have any effect on it. Once in existence it would never succumb to change and disappear or transform into something else. If the delusions in the mind of the sentient being who became the enlightened one of our era, Shakyamuni Buddha, were intrinsically established, how could he ever have got rid of them? How could 'elaborations,' meaning deluded conceptual minds, be stopped? If he inherently existed as a being in cyclic existence how could he have left it and entered the state beyond suffering? For him 'Nirvana would be impossible' (Verse 16). Not even the Buddhas, nor the *dharma*, nor the Sangha, none of the Three Jewels to which the Buddhist goes for refuge, exist from their own side.

Emptiness itself is also empty of inherent existence. Even some scholars within the Buddhist fold have held that emptiness has some absolute status beyond the interplay of dependent-arising. Emptiness is called ultimate truth, which might lead to the impression that is an absolute, objective reality transcending the relative. But this is far from being the case. The emptiness of inherent existence, for example, of a tree is called an ultimate truth because it is a phenomena such that, when it is perceived directly, the way it appears to the mind and the ways it actually exists are completely concordant. On the other hand a tree is called a conventional truth because it is a phenomena such that when it is perceived by anyone except a Buddha, the way it appears and the way it actually exists are not concordant, since a tree always appears to the mind of anyone who is not a Buddha to be inherently existent, but it is not. So emptiness is given the name 'ultimate' because the only consciousness that experiences it directly is one that has removed all the superimpositions of ignorance.

If we meditate deeply on the emptiness of the self and the objects of use of the self for a long period of time, gradually ignorance and the other delusions will be erased from our minds forever. Meditation on emptiness is the most powerful antidote for sufferings of cyclic existence there is, but of itself emptiness cannot do anything. From its own side it has no power or intention to relieve us of our sufferings. It is just one facet of the way things are. It is not something that anyone bows down to and worships. It is not an ultimate in the way that, for instance, the Christian God might perhaps be called "the ultimate one." It may be thought of it in terms of individual phenomena. We can reflect very fruitfully on the emptiness of a cup or a table for example. Just remembering that without a cup there would be no emptiness of inherent existence of a cup establishes that the emptiness of inherent existence of a cup is a dependent-arising, since it is dependent on the cup.

17

Therefore, who could challenge him
Who, in assemblies of the wise,
Has clearly proclaimed with lion's roar
Freedom from inherent nature?

18

Since lack of inherent nature
And the ability to function do not contradict,
Never mind that dependent-arising
And emptiness co-exist.

19

'By the reason of dependent-arising,
There are no ground for extreme views.'
For this fine teaching, O Protector,
Your speech is unexcelled.

20

'All is empty of self-nature!'
And, 'From this cause arises that effect!'
These two certainties assist each other
And abide in harmony.

21

What is more wonderful than this?
What is more marvellous than this?
If you are praised for this principle,
That is real praise, nothing else.

At the time the Buddha taught in India, many different schools of philosophy and many different esoteric mental disciplines which were supposed to be the key to liberation existed. Before these scholars and adepts listened to Buddha's teachings, none of them had hard about dependent-arising and emptiness, but once his teachings were revealed to them they had nothing which to rebut his formidable arguments in the 'assemblies of the wise' (verse 17). Some of Buddha's first disciples were famous teachers in their own right. Shariputra and Maudgalyayana were two whose followers are said to have numbered in the hundreds. When they heard Buddha's teachings, they proclaimed: 'By the reason of dependent-arising there are no grounds for extreme views' (verse 19) and 'All is empty of self-nature!' (verse 20), they found nothing to equal them in either profundity or extensiveness. When these noted teachers converted to Buddhism they brought their many followers with them, the twin ideas of dependent-arising and emptiness being the unique teachings of Buddha's system that won them over. Buddha's teaching that these two, dependent-arising and emptiness assist or mutually support each other is the principle of verse 21 that Buddha is worthy to be praised for above all else.

22

Those held in slavery by delusions,
Hopelessly resent you (so free and clear).
Small wonder that they find intolerable
That sound of, 'Non-inherent existence.'

23

But to accept dependent-arising,
The precious treasure of your speech,
Then resent the roar of emptiness;
This do I find surprising.

24

If through the very term of highest
Dependent-arising, the door that leads
To non-inherent existence, they grasp
Inherent existence, by what means

25

Can these people be led into
That good path which pleases you,
That incomparable entrance,
Well travelled by supreme Aryas?

There were also those who remained unattracted to Buddha's teachings. They are mentioned in verse 22 as being "held in slavery by delusions."

The followers of the one nihilistic, non-Buddhist, school were called Charvakas (Hedonists). Because they denied any validity to reasoning and denied past and future lives they were judged to have fallen to the extreme of nihilism. After the Buddhist view became well-known, other Hindu schools in India decided that there were now two schools that had veered to the extreme of nihilism, the Charvakas and the Buddhists! Even today there are scholars within the Indian tradition and also in the west who conclude that the Buddhists of the Consequentialist persuasion advance a completely nihilistic view. "Small wonder that they find intolerable/That sound of, 'non-inherent existence.'" It is not so surprising if those who do not have much understanding of dependent-arising reject what dependent-arising is supposed to prove, non-inherent existence, but that people who have studied dependent-arising and declare that they accept it should also spurn its natural consequence, emptiness–this Tsongkhapa does find contrary to expectations (verse 23). As we have seen, the stance of these thinkers, followers of the lower Buddhist schools, is to adhere to a rather more limited vision of dependent-arising. Buddha taught explicitly about emptiness in the *Perfect Wisdom Sutras*. The response of some of the followers of the two lowest schools, the Particularists and the Sutra followers, is to deny that these discourses were actually taught by the Buddha; and to say that the great clarifier of these teachings, Nagarjuna, does not deserve to be called a holder of the Buddhist view. Others from these two lower schools say that these discourses were only taught for small numbers of disciples and are not to be taken literally. The Mind Only followers and Autonomists accept the *Perfect Wisdom Sutra* as the Buddha's word, but also call them interpretive, rather than definitive scriptures, meaning that they should not be taken at face value; rather that the intended meaning is different from the apparent one.

Having arrived at the very gate of understanding non-inherent existence by having some understanding of dependent-arising then, these people fail to pass through the gate and follow the path which pleases the Buddhas. Those who follow this path are 'Aryas' (verse 25), that is, people who have realized emptiness directly and are in the process of applying the actual antidote to deluded ignorance by familiarising themselves single-pointedly with emptiness again and gain.

26

Inherent existence, unmade and non-dependent;
Dependently-related, made and dependent;
How can these two states be combined
On one base, without contradiction?

27

Therefore, whatever arises dependently
Though always free of inherent existence,
Appears to exist from its own side;
So you said this is like an illusion.

In this verse Buddha compares all phenomena to an illusion. Notice that he does not say all phenomena are illusions, merely that they are like illusions. The kind of illusion referred to by the Buddha is an illusion conjured up by an Indian magician of the type who is able to cause a pebble or a stick to appear as a horse or an elephant or as a handsome woman to his audience by casting a mantra that affects their eyes. The illusion appears to be a real horse, an elephant or woman but in truth, is not. Possibly this type of magician is not so common now as in the days of ancient India, although the modern day hypnotist is able to foster similar illusions in the minds of his subjects. But for a modern equivalent that will be within the direct experience of everyone we can use the example of images seen in films or on television. When children who are too young to understand the nature of the pictures that appear on television see what appears to be people, animals or food on a television screen they think these things are actually in space before them or inside the television. The way we apprehend these images is different. We readily associate them with the objects they represent but we do not grasp at them as being the actual objects. Sometimes when we watch television a very small image appears in the center of the screen, the image, say, of a car or a box of soap powder. The image grows bigger and bigger. This represents the object coming towards us. A young child or naive person who has never watched television before thinks that there is an object actually coming nearer to him. If we were asked if there was an object actually coming towards us, we would reply that of course there was not. Note, however, that although we are too sophisticated to take this illusion as real, even we can become so far immersed in the flickering images that we are filled now with fear, now with desire, mirth or sorrow.

The way ordinary people see phenomena is very similar to the way the young child sees the things that appear on television and to the way the magician's subjects see his illusory horse. The common factor is that in all three cases the viewer unconsciously superimposes onto the object viewed a mode of existence which the object does not possess. The image of a dog the child sees on television appears to be a real dog. The illusory horse is taken to be a real horse by those under the magician's spell. Objects, which are not inherently existent, appear to us to be inherently existent and we grasp at or assent to that appearance. When we who have both a strong appearance of inherent existence and a strong grasping at it hear for the first time that there is no such thing as inherent existence it may strike us as incredible. It runs very much counter to the view of the world that is ingrained in us and this appearance of inherent existence is no easy thing to dislodge. The water of a mirage on a road on a hot day persists in appearing as real water even when we know full well that is only an optical illusion caused by atmospheric conditions. Similarly even when Superior Beings, who are able to meditate on the emptiness of inherent existence single-pointedly and directly, arise from meditation they still have the appearance of phenomena as inherently existent. But one great difference between those Superior Beings and ordinary people is that the former do not assent to this deceptive appearance of inherent existence.

When an ordinary person sees an object such as a pair of shoes or a television in a shop window, the object in the first place appears to that being's eye consciousness as inherently existent. Then in the case where the person becomes attracted to the object, his discrimination that the object is desirable and his subsequent wish to possess it are induced and strengthened up by the mind which grasps at the object to exist from its own side. In this frame of mind, the person grasps that the object's ability to give the owner of it happiness is intrinsic to the object. The object's gleaming, brand-new appearance makes it particularly appealing. If we think about it, even this aspect is grasped at as inherent in the object, and not discounted as something that will have vanished in the first week of use. Beyond that there is a third level of being affected by the superimposed factor of inherent existence. This occurs when the person actually takes possession of the object. At this time the attachment induced by grasping the object to be inherently existent and inherently pleasant mixes with attachment which arises from thinking, 'This object is mine,' while grasping the self to be inherently existent. We can also describe how the feeling of hatred towards, say, someone whom we discriminate as an enemy, first arises and then intensifies to an altogether exaggerated degree in three stages: firstly the stage of the mere appearance of inherent existence; secondly, the stage of assenting to and grasping at that appearance and thereupon generating hatred; and thirdly the stage of very strong hatred when grasping at our own self as inherently existent comes into the equation as well. In the train of these strong delusions come deluded actions. Through attachment we indulge in acts of miserliness or violence to clutch on to our possessions. Out of hatred we descend to abuse, slander, scorn and far, far worse.

Superior or Arya Beings (as we said, those who have seen emptiness directly), with the exception of Buddhas, still have the first of the above three stages, in which phenomena appear to them as inherently existent, but they are not deceived by this appearance. They know that it is in truth an illusion, so they are at the point where they can abandon engaging in actions which perpetuate the cycle of death and rebirth. They do not develop delusions in dependence upon the appearance of inherent existence, and not generating these delusions they do not engage in negative actions. For this reason they do not create new causes to be reborn in cyclic existence. There is a further development when a Superior of the Great Vehicle lineage attains Buddhahood. Not only does a Buddha Superior not grasp at things as inherently existent, but, it is said, at that time things cease even to appear as inherently existent to him. What does a being who has reached the state of the highest enlightenment see then? It is said that the Buddha does not see conventional truths, that is, the phenomena of the world, such as house, clouds and trees from his own point of view. Rather, he understands the appearance of these conventional phenomena from the point of view of ordinary beings. He is said to apprehend conventional phenomena simply by knowing what ordinary beings are experiencing. This is an explanation which may well sound inconceivable when we first hear it. Our ordinary understanding finds it difficult to expand far enough to encompass a Buddha's surpassing qualities of realization and compassionate action. Only a Buddha is said to be able to fully comprehend the good qualities of a Buddha. Nevertheless, explanations of how phenomena are like an illusion, in appearing to exists inherently while not so existing, are within the scope of reasoning, and, in spite of some people's initial reaction to these teachings as far-fetched and fanciful, if we think about them carefully we will come to see that in the end the only way any phenomena can possibly exist is as a dependent-arising, devoid of intrinsic identity.

28

Through this very fact we can well understand
The assertion that, in the way you taught,
Those who would challenge you
By way of logic can find no fallacy.

29

Why? Because your explanation
Makes remote the chance that one
Will exaggerate or deny
Manifest or non-manifest things.

30

Your speech is seen as peerless
Because it presents the path of dependent-arising,
And this gives rise to certainty
That (your) other teachings are valid too.

Thus, as it implies in verse 28, the one who can overturn the Buddha's teachings on the way things exist has not yet been born. On the philosophical side of the teachings Buddhism takes its stand squarely on logic and reasoning. That is why the Buddha's teachings offer such a clear path of mental development. In verse 29 'manifest' and 'non-manifest' things refers to phenomena that we can experience directly with our senses and to phenomena that we can only initially comprehend by using reasoning, respectively. These two categories between them cover all phenomena. Exaggerating phenomena means ascribing to them a mode of existence that they do not have. Denying them means not recognizing a mode of existence that they do in fact possess. We can investigate for ourselves whether the teachings on emptiness and dependent-arising are true or not using our reasoning powers. Other aspects of the Buddha's teachings are less amenable to reasoning, for instance his teaching that generosity in this life leads one to enjoy resources in future lives and the practice of ethical behaviour in this life leads one to enjoy happiness in future lives. In verse 30 Tsongkhapa indicates that directly realizing emptiness as he did will inspire such a respect for the insight of the teacher who taught it that one will have great confidence that those other less easily verifiable aspects of the Buddha's teachings are true too.

31

You saw reality, and taught it well.
Those who train in your footsteps
Will transcend all troubles,
For they shall destroy the root of evil.

32

But those who turn away from your teaching,
Though they wearily struggle, long and hard,
Invite problems, one after the other,
By their firm views of a self.

33

Marvellous! When the wise comprehend
The difference between these two (trainings),
How can they fail to respect you
From their innermost hearts?

The next set of verses, 31 to 33, compares the prospects of those who follow in the footsteps of the Buddha and those who look elsewhere for direction. Seeing what the Buddha saw about the way things exist does not simply bring about the abstract satisfaction of finding out something that happens to be true, but it means that one has at last arrived at a view which is contradictory to and can displace the deep-rooted grasping at a self of persons and phenomena, the deceptive perspective which leads us again and again into harming others and bringing all suffering on to ourselves. Without identifying this deeply embedded misunderstanding about the self as the fundamental source of all our troubles any other attempts to find happiness will only be treating the symptoms of the disease rather than the source of it. As we have already suggested to try to describe what the Buddha saw when he 'saw reality' (verse 31) is extremely difficult. One more clue we can take account of is that Buddha and only a Buddha can see a phenomena's conventional and ultimate nature simultaneously. This signifies for instance that he sees both a cup and the emptiness of inherent existence of that cup together at the same time. People who have realized emptiness directly but who have not reached Buddhahood can observe either the conventional nature or the ultimate one, not both simultaneously.

When we try to conceive of the experience of realizing just the ultimate nature of an object such as a cup or the self, it may be helpful in terms of an analogy to think about empty space. This phenomena has some similarities with emptiness in the way it appears to the mind. Both these phenomena are permanent, which means they are static and not changing from moment to moment in a causal series. Both are understood only in terms of there being an absence of some other phenomena. The meaning of space or uncaused space is lack of obstruction and contact. Due to there being an underlying absence of obstruction and contact, forms that occupy space such as houses, our bodies and cups have room to exist in the place they do. Due to there being empty space in a cup, it can be filled with something such as tea. But this lack of obstruction and contact does not have any implied qualities. The absence of a coin in our hand is similar. Such a phenomena is only cognized by bringing our idea of a coin to mind, looking for one in the hand and then negating it. In the same way we can only understand emptiness by first of all bringing our idea of inherent existence to mind, searching for it and then negating it. Although we grasp at objects to be inherently existent all the time, it requires plenty of thought about dependent-arising before we can single out the superimposed aspect of inherent existence. This we must do with exact precision before we can negate it and meditate on its absence. So, as when cognizing empty space, one is essentially cognizing a lack of something when one perceives emptiness. In the latter case it is the absence of something whose existence one formerly took for granted. To say that an experience of emptiness is like having a vision of light or something like that could be misleading therefore, in that light, being form, has positive qualities, whereas emptiness is only a state of negation. One person in Tibet went around proclaiming that he had realized emptiness. He was asked to describe it and he said it was like a pigeon. After that he was given the nickname, Professor Pigeon! But, from what other people say, we can suggest that when one experiences emptiness one experiences a very relaxed sort of feeling. Due to our delusions, our mind is in a state of constant agitation, like boiling water. Disturbing states of mind are constantly arising; conceptions and projections bubble up endlessly. When one realizes emptiness it is as though someone pours a large amount of cold water onto that boiling water, which then becomes cool and very still. The mind becomes relaxed and clear in a way it never has been before. We should not be discouraged by thinking that emptiness is very difficult to realize correctly. We should do all we can to understand it even on a very gross level because this will plant imprints on our minds to realize it more precisely in the future. Finally, in order to realize emptiness and see reality we cannot neglect the other aspects of the path, such as training in ethical conduct, loving kindness, concentration and so on. These help to purify, energize and inspire the mind to focus powerfully on the subtleties of the correct view.

34

Not to mention the entire wealth of your teachings,
Just generally understanding
One small part of them,
Is to bring supreme bliss.

35

Alas! My own mind was ruled by confusion
When long ago I sought refuge,
Blind to your teachings' vast qualities,
Not to mention their fine details.

36

Yet the stream of life has not yet sunk
Into the mouth of the Lord of Death,
And I have a little belief in you.
Even this I think fortunate.

However, if we did only have a chance to understand 'one small part' of the teachings, the part that would bring supreme bliss above all is the teachings on dependent-arising.This is how we can interpret verse 34. Verses 35 and 36 strike a more personal note. Tsongkhapa relates how little he understood of the Buddha's teachings when first he went for refuge. But now, having finally gained a deep understanding of the essence of the Buddha's wisdom, he is able to see exactly why Buddha is the ultimate refuge. Even though Tsongkhapa is revered as one of the very greatest scholars and adepts who reinvigorated and clarified the Buddhist doctrine in Tibet and left behind a magnificent corpus of writings including commentaries of the most penetrating kind, it seems that when he is compared to the Buddha himself, the Buddha's qualities are vaster still. If we stand by the side of an extensive lake the expanse of water may seem enormous, but in comparison to it the waters of an ocean are far wider and still deeper.

VIII

CONCLUSION

37

Of teachers, the teacher of dependent-arising,
Of wisdom, the wisdom of dependent-arising;
Like kings over all conquerors in the world,
These prove your wisdom supreme.

The Buddha's unique qualities that made his appearance in this world-system inestimably valuable were his possessing the wisdom of dependent-arising and his teaching of it. Otherwise ones preceded the Buddha or appeared subsequently, but if they had any understanding of dependent-arising they failed to teach it to a wide audience, or if on the other hand, they were eloquent and skilful teachers, they lacked wisdom and had nothing to say about dependent-arising. Having the teachings on dependent-arising still available together with the wisdom realizing those teachings is said to be like still enjoying the Buddha's presence in our world today.

38

All that you have taught
is related to dependent-arising;
And since this leads to Nirvana,
No deed of yours does not bring peace.

39

Wonderful is your teaching!
Since whoever listens
Will attain peace, who could not
Be devoted to preserving such teachings?

40

As it overcomes all opponents,
Is free from internal contradictions
And fulfils both goals of beings,
My delight ever grows for this Doctrine.

Even though the teachings of the Buddha are very extensive, in terms of the range of subjects covered and thoroughness with which they are explained all of them relate directly or indirectly to the profound dependent-arising, since this is the very essence of them. As we have reviewed a few of the differences between the four different tenet systems that have been codified from the great collection of teachings, we have noted teachings that are quite contradictory to one another. In one place Buddhism allowed that the self inherently exists. In another he refuted inherent existence with abundant reasons. This is but a variety of approaches to the one goal of leading beings of all different aptitudes to an unmistaken understanding of the full meaning of dependent-arising at its deepest level. For instance, there was a king called Ajata-shatru who ruled over a certain part of India at the time of the Buddha. He was so evil that he had even murdered his own father and mother in order to gain the throne for himself. His way of life was therefore utterly contrary to the one that Buddha was teaching. He developed a strong antipathy towards the Buddha and tried to kill him too, once by sending a mad elephant charging towards where the Buddha was teaching in the hope that he might be trampled to death. This king rejected the idea that there were any higher beings who could be an object of refuge for people. He rejected the necessity for practising virtue and also the existence of past and future lives. However, his mother and father had great faith in the Buddha and they both had led virtuous lives. The father had spoken to his son many times about the Buddha's teachings. When he was killed he was reborn in a celestial realm. He then showed himself in the form a deity to his son. His son received a great shock when this happened and his former materialistic outlook was completely overturned. He saw that there were past and future lives and became very afraid of the future consequences of having killed his mother and father. The king decided to go to the Buddha and throw himself at his feet. The Buddha was aware of this and knew that if he told the king, once he had made his confession, how intensely negative the act of killing one's parents is, then the king would be plunged into such great despair that he might even die from it. The Buddha therefore understood that on this occasion telling the bald truth would not be beneficial. So what the Buddha said to the king was that in order to practise *dharma* the first thing one should do is to kill one's mother and father. Then one should kill the king of the kingdom, then his two chief ministers, all his attendants, than all the servants of the attendants. The king was extremely fascinated by this teaching and was amazed that the Buddha should have taught it. With his overwhelming anxiety about his actions diverted in this way, the king was able to think more clearly, and, back in his palace, he pondered what the Buddha had said. He understood the Buddha to be a person who had abandoned violence in all its form, yet here he was teaching that one should kill people in order to find liberation from suffering. The king pondered further and eventually reached the understanding that the superficial level of the teaching was device to trap his attention, while on another level killing one's father and mother referred to destroying the root ignorance and the *karma* which springs from that ignorance. Ignorance and *karma* lead to rebirth in cyclic existence. In this way they are like the father and mother from whom all beings in cyclic existence are born. Killing the king of the kingdom refers to eliminating the states of mind which instigate actions that cause rebirth in cyclic existence. The mind is the instigator of all unskilful actions and within the context of a person, the mind is like the king in a kingdom. These three elements, ignorance, *karma* and consciousness are the first three of the twelve links of dependent-arising. The two chief ministers that have to be killed can either be interpreted as two more of the twelve links or as the two extremes, the views of permanence and nihilism. The rest of the twelve links are what is referred to by the royal attendants. Then the servants of the attendants refers to all the objects in cyclic existence. So the Buddha's implicit teaching was that if one eliminates all these, one will attain liberation, by bringing the production of the twelve links of dependent-arising to a halt. By the time King Ajatashatru had deduced all this, a great faith in the Buddha had awakened in him and he went on to become one of the major patrons of the Buddha in those days. This is one example of the way in which Buddha had a special ability to guide beings with different dispositions along different paths to a full understanding of dependent-arising. It also shows how 'internal contradictions' (verse 40) between different teachings that are apparent on the superficial level are resolved when their full import becomes clear.

Also in verse 40, the two 'goals of beings' that the Buddha's teachings fulfils are the goals of oneself and of others. The Buddha is not just someone who has achieved peace for himself but has also perfected his capacity to bring others to peace. He does not just teach the path to individual liberation but also the more arduous stages of evolving to the higher state of complete enlightenment for the benefit of all. Just how difficult and long this second path can be is indicated in verse 41.

41

For the sake of the Doctrine you gave
Again and again over countless aeons,
Sometimes your body, sometimes your life,
Your dear family, and treasures of wealth.

The path to full enlightenment is called the way of a bodhisattva. A bodhisattva is someone who is dedicated to achieving Buddhahood for all beings. His understanding of emptiness has to be more extensive than that of someone going to individual liberation and also the bodhisattva must accumulate a far vaster store of virtues, serving the welfare of others over and over again for countless lifetimes.

In the last section of *Praise for Dependent-Arising* before the concluding verses Tsongkhapa reveals some of his personal experiences in trying to follow this very path of the bodhisattva warrior. No individual dramatic acts of self-sacrifice are recorded, but the picture of a life of unswerving dedication is conveyed by the string of illuminating images. They describe the uplift of energy and the protection from sorrow which flow from pure faith in one's teacher and the blissful relief of finally coming to the actual quintessential meaning of the teachings, the experience which inspired these words. And if anyone should ask about Tsongkhapa's efforts on behalf of other sentient beings, we have only to point to his teachings, such as this *Praise* itself, as evidence of his lifelong devotion to helping others by transmitting to them the Buddha's speech and thus inspiring them to abandon sorrow.

42

When I contemplate the excellences of your Dharma,
You appear to my mind
As a fish is drawn by the hook;
How sad my fate to have not heard it from you.

43

The intensity of this sadness
Does not let my mind go free,
Just as a mother's mind never separates
From the thought of her beloved, lost child.

44

But when I reflect on your speech, thinking,
'Blazing with splendour of holy mark and signs,
Haloed by rays of light,
O Teacher, with your beautiful Brahma voice,

45

You spoke in this way,' then in my mind
The image of Shakyamuni arises and
Immediately my sorrows are healed,
As moonbeams sooth a fever.

The first of the series of images describes how he is captivated by the good qualities of the *dharma* like a fish hooked tight, but feels a piercing sadness at not having heard the teachings from the Buddha himself. Through great faith, the Buddha appears instead to his mind's eyes, splendidly arrayed, discoursing in a melodious voice. A circle of disciples was fortunate enough to be present when the Buddha turned the wheel of *dharma* in person. Visualizing himself as one of those, he receives blessings which dissolve his sorrows. Tsongkhapa compares these blessings to moonbeams which are able to soothe the torment of heat. In a country like India the days can be oppressively hot, but when the moon comes out in the evening, its rays seem to have a pacifying, cooling effect. People are sensitive to moonlight in different ways however. A few people find the moon's influence disturbing. It makes them restless and unable to sleep, even very lively.

46

Although this good system is so marvellous,
The unskilled become totally confused.
Ideas all tangled in every way,
Just like balbaza grass.

47

Having understood the problem, I then
Schooled myself (in the texts of) skilled sages,
And with energy listened here and there,
Ever seeking the meaning of your intention.

48

I studied many treatises
Of Buddhist and non-Buddhist schools,
Yet my mind was tormented sorely,
Time and again in the web of doubt.

49

Nagarjuna was prophesied, to explain rightly
The principle of your final vehicle,
Free from the extremes of existence and non-existence.
When I, through the kindness of the lama,

50

Beheld the night-lily garden of his treatises
Illuminated by garlands of white light,
True eloquence of the glorious Moon (Chandrakirti),
Whose bright orb of immaculate wisdom

51

Moves freely across the sky of scripture,
Dispelling the darkness of extremist hearts
And outshining the constellations of wrong speech,
My mind found relief at last.

From the faith indicated in verses 42 to 45 arose Tsongkhapa's unquenchable enthusiasm for study. Some details of how he studied occupy the next group of verses (46 to 51). In the history of Buddhism many great beings have taken birth and have extracted from the Buddha's teachings various philosophical systems suitable to the people present at a particular time and place. Some notable names are Asanga, Nagarjuna, Bhavaviveka and Buddhapalita who were the great pioneers of the Mind-Only view, the Middle Way view, the view of the Autonomist branch of the Middle Way School and the view of the Consequentialist branch of that school respectively. The followers of these teachers were then led into many different debates on the finer points of the teachings. However a newcomer to the Buddha's philosophy could not be expected to develop much curiosity about these disputes straight away without seeing the reason for them. He perhaps would see all the different ideas tangled together, like balbaza grass (verse 46), a sort of grass that grows in India, a similar plant being found in Tibet as well. It grows in huge, densely interwind clumps and can cause irritation to the skin. On the other hand, when one develops a lot of doubts and has a desire to ask a lot of questions about the Buddhist view, then this is regarded as a favourable sign. It indicates that one has sufficient curiosity and application to make one's own attempt on these lofty peaks of wisdom. The highest, Consequentialist, view has been clearly set forth but it is said that only those of sharp intelligence can understand Buddha's ultimate intent by studying his ultimate view alone, and passively to acquiesce in the highest view, merely because our teacher says it is the highest view is not something even those who incline to 'Buddhism of the heart' rather than 'Buddhism of the head' should really be content with. It is as if Buddha deliberately delivered teachings open to different levels of interpretation in order to provoke his followers into debating one side of a question against another. In doing so we will refine and sharpen our minds to the level where we can begin to understand the truth's vital subtleties and further more we will then arrive at the correct conclusions actively, through our own power of reasoning. Thus the truth will not remain as a dogma to which we feebly assent, but will become a powerful force vanquishing confusion, bestowing clarity, and efficacious for good.

Tsongkhapa certainly studied the writings of the lower Buddhist schools, only to be left dissatisfied and unconvinced by their presentations (verse 48). Nonetheless his study of the lower Buddhist schools and his identification of their defects would be an entirely suitable preparation for his deeper sounding of the Consequentialist view. In one of the most beautiful metaphors of the 'Praise' (verse 49-51) , he describes how he studied the Consequentialist view mainly through the texts of Nagarjuna and Chandrakirti. Tsongkhapa wrote the *Praise for Dependent-Arising* out of his own thorough realization of the final view, and his guides for the last part of the journey to that goal were these two geniuses. Nagarjuna blazed the trail to be followed by those upholding the view that emptiness and dependent-arising are non-contradictory. Chandrakirti drew forth the meaning of Nagarjuna's texts and explained the distinctive features of the Consequentialist view very clearly. Nagarjuna's treatises are likened to a night-lily garden(verse 49). Night-lilies are so called because they are said to bloom only at night, by the light of the moon.

Thus Chandrakirti, the first part of whose name means moon, is likened to the moon which bathes the garden in white light and causes the flowers of the night-lilies to open and reveal their beauties. Earlier Tsongkhapa compared the blessings that come from visualizing the Buddha to the soothing radiance of the moon. Here (verse 51) he describes how he find final relief by opening his heart to the moonbeams of pure wisdom which dispels completely the darkness of misunderstanding. Immediately he mentions the kindness of his guru, or personal teacher in guiding him to such a state of freedom.

Nagarjuna composed six texts explaining emptiness and setting out the Middle Way view. The emphasis in them is strongly on refuting the view grasping at inherent existence which was prevalent amongst the students of Buddhism of his day. Nagarjuna was both a renowned scholar and a practitioner and his texts were much studied. Opponents who were unable to discriminate between no existence and no inherent existence were quick to accuse him of denying the existence of phenomena altogether. Chandrakirti replied to these critics by setting forth not just the way in which phenomena are devoid of inherent existence but also the way in which they do none the less conventionally exist. Having exposed the error of acquiescing in the illusory appearance of inherent existence he proceeds to dwell on the dependently related mode of existence that phenomena do actually have. Those who are interested in finding out more about the Middle Way view should study this text, *Supplement to the Middle Way*. This would be the best introduction to Nagarjuna's works.

At the time of Tsongkhapa also there were considerable disagreement about how the view of the

Middle Way should be exactly understood. Tsongkhapa received a vision of Manjushri, the deity who is the embodiment of all the Buddha's wisdom, symbolized by the flaming sword he holds aloft. In answer to Tsongkhapa's request for guidance, Manjushri directed him to rely on Chandrakirit's *Supplement to the Middle Way* as a faultless exposition by one who had complete understanding. After he had completed his own purpose by dispelling the perplexity of wrong views in his own mind, Tsongkhapa in turn composed many works which have kept the ancient flame of Buddha's profoundest wisdom burning purely for the generations who have come after him. Tsongkhapa's life was short compared to Buddha's and Nagarjuna's but he left a treasure house of commentaries and expositions of the scriptures behind. Like the Buddha we should not praise him for his realizations alone, but also for the eloquence and skill with which he offered his surpassing knowledge to others.

52

Of all his deeds, Buddha's speech is supreme,
And, for this very reason, true sages
Should commemorate the Perfect One
For this (teaching on dependent-arising).

In verse 52, Tsongkhapa singles out Buddha's 'speech,' i.e., his teaching, as his supreme deed, because this is the action which has benefitted sentient beings the most. Buddha is credited with having performed many miracles. For instance the adepts of some other Indian paths of knowledge disputed with Buddha some time after his enlightenment and engaged him in a contest of magical powers. Buddha won the contest, but where are those magical emanations and those other yogis now? When we see paintings of the miracles Buddha performed we may wonder whether these things really happened or not. In any case these fabulous deeds are lost in the past, while his teachings on the other hand are still very much with us, preserved in a pure form of words and in the minds of those with realizations.

53

Inspired by the teacher, I renounced the world
And studied well the Conqueror's teaching
I have been diligent in yoga practice, such is
This monk's reverence for the Great Seer.

54

By the kindness of my guru I was fortunate to meet
The liberating teaching of the peerless guide,
Therefore I dedicate this virtue as a cause
For all beings to be received by spiritual friends.

55

Until samsara ends, may the beneficent one's teaching
Be undisturbed by the winds of wrong views;
May all beings in the world forever understand
The essence of the teachings, and have faith in the teacher.

56

May they uphold Shakyamuni's excellent way,
Which reveals the principle of dependent-arising.
Through all their lives let them never waver,
Even at the cost of their bodies, or their lives.

57

Day and night may they always be thinking
How to best propagate this glorious success
Achieved by the Supreme Liberator, in lives
Of assiduous effort beyond measure.

58

When beings strive with pure intention (to preserve this Doctrine)
May Brahma, Indra and the world protectors,
And the guardians, such as Mahakala,
Be constant aides, never letting them down.

These remaining six verses bring the *Praise for Dependent-Arising* to its conclusion with a prayer for auspiciousness. In verse 53 and 54 Tsongkhapa still has a little more to say about his own personal journey on the Buddhist path, of his renunciation of the world, which led him to become a monk, and of his 'yoga practice.' We should understand that not only did Tsongkhapa engage with an extraordinary degree of effort in the study of philosophy but he also did not neglect the esoteric side of Buddha's teachings. As with most of the great masters in the Tibetan tradition of Buddhism it would be a mistake to think of Tsongkhapa as only a philosopher, however distinguished; he was thoroughly versed in all aspects of Buddhist practice.

In verse 53 he pays reverence to the Buddha under the title of the Great Seer (Maharishi). This epithet of the Buddha goes back to the days before he became enlightened, to the time when he spent six years seeking that state through the practice of physical austerity. It was a path he eventually rejected but not before impressing his fellow ascetics so much with his practices of fasting, long periods of sitting upright in meditation and other forms of self-denial that they gave him the title of Great Seer. The literal meaning of the word *Rishi* (rendered *drang srong* in Tibetan) includes the senses 'honest' or 'upright' and 'to straighten.' It applies to holy men who give up worldly life, live by begging and follow a spiritual path based on physical hardship and abstinence. In the next verse Tsongkhapa again reminds the reader who might be inspired to become interested in Buddhism for the first time of the supreme importance of a personal teacher or spiritual guide. It cannot all be learned from books! Indebted as he is to the kindness of his own lama, he prays that any virtue that has been created through composing this praise may act as a cause for all beings to come under the indispensable care of such a personal teacher. Next he prays that the virtue may go in some way to protect all beings from wrong views and bestow correct understanding (verse 55). He prays that they may uphold the key principle of dependent-arising in any adversity and cause it to flourish throughout the worlds (verses 56 and 57). Finally he calls upon the worldly gods such as Brahma and Indra, upon the world protectors and the sworn protector deities of Buddhism such as Mahakala, requesting that they also do their share to spread the teachings of the Enlightened One.

If we are to derive benefit from the Buddha's teachings, in fulfilment of the spirit in which they were given, then we have to develop an interest in examining our own mind, for beyond all the other more superficial causes of enjoyment and suffering, our mind is the ultimate deciding factor in whether we are happy or not. One pre-eminent feature of the mind is that it can be trained. It tends to respond to the objects it meets in the ways it is familiar with, but can be accustomed, not always quickly, to more constructive and beneficial responses. If we find that our impulsive desires keep leading us into conflict with others and to dissatisfaction with ourselves, it is time to start examining more thoroughly where we expect those desires to lead us. We should look ahead to what the results are likely to be if those desires are indulged. If it looks in the long terms as though there is likely to be more benefit than harm caused, all well and good. What is often the case however is that we grasp at the short-term results of our actions, scarcely stopping to consider the long-term cost, either to ourselves or others. If we can create within ourselves a degree of mental freedom such that we do not become totally involved in our desires without thinking through the consequences first, then we will be making progress. Or take an unpleasant state of mind like being strongly jealous of someone. Practising the *dharma* can certainly eliminate such negative moods. Studying the dharma should in the first place lead us to see that it is an irrational state of mind that benefits nobody and that there are far more wholesome objects of our attention than the object of our resentment. But of course our approach has to be a balanced one. While trying to change ourselves for the better we have to accept who we are at any particular stage, without developing aversion towards our own thoughts because we cannot get rid of strong negative states of mind immediately.

When our jealousy is aroused there is not much we can do other than try to avoid being in the presence of the person who is acting as the magnet for these feelings. We have to try in whichever way we can to avoid that person. When the jealousy dies down, as it surely will, we can examine it more easily. Many of the explanations of dependent-arising and emptiness we have offered through the course of this book are very much applicable in reducing such a negative emotion. Gradually, through thinking about and discussing them we will understand how to apply them. Or, in the case of being jealous of someone because of their greater cleverness and better educational qualifications, for instance we can think 'If I become jealous of this person because they are cleverer than me, how will it benefit me? Being jealous does not lead me to have those qualities I desire. As for the effect on the other person, it neither helps nor harms him. All I am doing is bringing unhappiness on myself without any advantage at all.' Basically, in a case like this, we should aim not just to act on reasons that occur to us on the spur of the moment and fall into an all too familiar ugly mood or an unsuitable pattern of behaviour. We have to try to be objective in our examination of our motives and then we should think of as many of the negative effects of such a mood or behaviour as we can. If we are thorough about making the above investigation but still we feel we cannot trust our own judgement then perhaps we need to rely on the more objective judgement of others who are more highly developed than ourselves in their understanding of the mind. All this time, if we study the Buddha's teachings in general and try to put them into practice, then our own understanding will gradually become clearer and our ability to examine our own minds more sure.

The most important thing of all to understand is dependent-arising. In the short or medium-term Buddha's teachings can bring peace of mind in terms of being able to deal with the problems we encounter in going about everyday lives, but we should keep the long-term goal of completely realizing dependent-arising in mind. We should try to approach the understanding of it in two ways, firstly by accumulating a store of meritorious energy and ridding ourselves of previously accumulated negative energy and secondly by studying and meditating on dependent-arising, becoming more and more familiar with the ways of analysing we have explained.

Accumulating merit and eliminating negativities comes under the heading of the practice of ethics which is the first of three higher trainings mentioned earlier. A monk or nun has vows to keep. There are also vows that can be taken by lay people. Otherwise one should use the list of ten non-virtuous and ten virtuous actions to guide one's behaviour. The ten non-virtuous actions to be avoided are killing, stealing, sexual misconduct, lying, slander, harsh words, idle gossip, covetousness, wishing to harm and wrong views. The ten virtuous actions consist in definitely and deliberately not doing any of the ten non-virtues. This ethical training, over time, makes a stable and firm base of the mind and gives a chance of success to our efforts in the other two trainings of concentration and wisdom. One has to practice both of these trainings, though traditionally it is said that if one has less time one should practice the training of concentration more, whereas if one has more time to study in depth, then the training in wisdom is what one should emphasize.

Training in concentration involves developing the mind to the point where it can stay focused single-pointedly on any chosen object without wavering or becoming tired. This state is called calm-abiding. We choose a single object of meditation, such as the image of a particular Buddha, and practise placing the mind on that object again and again, only for short sessions in the beginning, but for longer and longer as time goes on. Between sessions of this type of meditation we should consider the disadvantages of cyclic existence, what causes it and how to escape from it. At other times we should think about the nature of the 'I' and the ways in which it does and does not exist. If we mix our meditations together like this, we will ensure that our practice has a certain breadth and scope. Those of us who have more time to dwell on the training of wisdom take more teachings and study more texts, but still mix these activities with our own analysis and meditation. We should take care that the text we use are authentic ones written by those who are skilled in the subject, because anything good always has its shoddy imitations. We should not dismiss the views of the lower schools, but rather practise trying to see things from their perspectives. Sharpening our mind on subtle impermanence and selflessness as put forward in the lower schools' systems is an excellent preparation for cutting through the unequalled Consequentialist insights. In meditation we can start with the lowest school and try to work up to the view of the highest school. It is also very useful to perform this type of meditation in reverse order, starting off with the most subtle object of refutation and working down the scale to the grossest.

Whatever *dharma* practice we engage in, whether it is practising analytical meditation based on reasoning, or placement meditation, where one focuses the mind only on one object, whether one is practising moral discipline, or accumulating merit by helping others, what one should never do is eagerly expect some marvellous effect in just a short time. 'Abandon the hope of results' is excellent advice. Grasping at achieving *dharma* realizations is a sure way to prevent them occurring and can lead to all sorts of false pride or despondency. We should try to strive to do our best and attain the goals that Buddha talked about without having fixed ideas about when we hope to achieve anything. What we need is a stable and firm type of practice. What we have in our minds at the moment are very firm and stable tendencies towards various delusions. When we practise *dharma* we try to build up predispositions towards virtuous states of mind and towards wisdom. If we practise well over a long period of time then these latter kinds of predispositions will become stable and strong. If someone carved a Buddha image out of a boulder, then we would expect it to last for a long time. On the other hand if he or she simply painted a Buddha image on the rock, less effort would be involved but the rain and the other elements would soon get to work and destroy it. In our *dharma* practice we should aim to be like the person who sculptures the stone, making the extra effort required to bring forth a Buddha out of the rough rock by patient chiselling, for the sake of a more enduring result.

Even though the seeds of delusion sprout profusely in our minds at the moment, since these delusions are based on misunderstanding of reality, they cannot after all be impossible to get rid of. As soon as we achieve a clear understanding, our ignorance must give way like darkness before light. The predispositions we place on our mindstream when we meditate on dependent-arising are very stable because they are based on reality. So even if these predispositions do not ripen up into a realization of dependent-arising in this lifetimes, because they are based on the truth and have some stability, there is every reason to hope they will ripen up in a future existence. Then, by prolonged acquaintance with and meditation on this precious realization of dependent-arising our delusions can be uprooted once and for all. Confident then, that the results of practising these teachings of the Enlightened One, passed down through Nagarjuna, Chandrakirit and Tsongkhapa will be very beneficial, we should enter into the practice of them with a relaxed and happy attitude. When we become more deeply acquainted with them we may reach the conclusion that there is nothing whatever more beneficial than them for sentient beings, in which case we will approach them in a mood of gladness and rejoicing. Howsoever, a feeling of pleasure when practising the *dharma* is worth a great deal. There are various reasons why we might be inclined to take these teachings very seriously; because they are very profound and need plenty of careful thought; because they are the gateway to the highest wisdom; because they precipitate a fundamental change of heart in us towards the allurements of cyclic existence. Nonetheless a tight or tense mind will only be a hindrance, so we should keep a happy mind at the beginning, in the middle and at the end.

BIBLIOGRAPHY

TIBETAN AND SANSKRIT WORKS

Āryadeva ('phags pa lha, second to third century C.E.)
The Four Hundred: Treatise of the Four Hundred Stanzas
Catuhsatakasastrakarika
Bstan bcos bzhi brgya pa zhes bya ba'i tshig le'ur byas pa

Chandrakirt (zla ba grags pa, seventh century)
Supplement to the Middle Way/ Supplement to (Nagarjuna's) Treatise on Middle way.
Madhyamakavatara
Dbu ma la 'jug pa
English translation (Ch. I-V): Jeffrey Hopkins in *Compassion in Tibetan Buddhism*, Valois, NY: Gabriel Snow Lion, 1980.
English translation (Ch. VI): Stepehen Batchelor in Geshe Rabten's *Echoes of Voidness*. London: Wisdom, 1982.

Dharmakirti (chos kyi grags pa, seventh century)
Commentary on Valid Cognition/ Commentary on (Dignaga's) Compendium on Valid Cognition.
Pramanavartikakarika
Tshad ma rnam 'grel gyi tshig le'ur byas pa

Nagarjuna (klu sgrub, first to second century CE)
Treatise on the Middle Way/ Fundamental Treatise on the Middle Way, Called 'Wisdom'
Madhyamasastra/Prajnanamamulamadhyamaka-karika

Dbu ma's bstan bcos/dbu ma rtsa ba'i tshig le'ur byas pa shes rab ces bya ba

English translation: David J. Kalupahana, *Nagarjuna: The Philosophy of the Middle Way*. Albany: State University Press of New York, 1986.

Tsongkhapa 1357-1419)

The Essence of Eloquent Sppech: Treatise Distinguishing the Interpretable and the Definitive
Drang ba dang nges pa'i don rnam par phye ba'i bstan bcos legs bshad snying po.

English Translation: Robert Thurman, *Tsong Khapa's Speech of Gold in the Essence of True Eloquence'*. Princeton, Princetòn University Press, 1984. Reprint, Delhi: Motilal Banarsidass, 1989.

OTHER WORKS

Hopkins, Jeffrey, *Meditation on Emptiness*. London: Wisdom, 1983.

Thurman, Robert, *Tsong Khapa's Speech of Gold in the 'Essence of True Eloquence'*. Princeton: Princeton University Press, 1984. Reprint, Delhi: Motilal Banarsidass, 1989.

OTHER BOOKS BY VEN. LOBSANG GYATSO

MAJOR WORKS

	Titles	*Language*
1.	The Magic Key of Eloquent Sayings -Pt. I	Tibetan
2.	The Magic Key of Eloquent Sayings -Pt. 2	Tibetan
3.	Jewel Treasure (on Tibetan grammar)	Tibetan
4.	Types of Mind and Mental Factors (*blo-rig*)	Tibetan
5.	The Three Objects of Refuge and *karma*	Tibetan
6.	Bod-kyi dul-thig (Truth about Tibetan the Tibetan issue)	Tibetan
7.	The Essence of Madhyamaka Philosophy	Tibetan
8.	Cultivating Bodhicitta	Tibetan
9.	Mirror of Kongtse-rapa	Tibetan
10.	Sunny Essence (Commentary to *Praise for Dependent-Arising*)	Tibetan
11.	Auspicious Opening (Union of Politics and Religion)	Tibetan
12.	Golden Spoon - Fundamentals of Buddhism	Tibetan
13.	The Tibetan Dhammapada	English
14.	The Harmony of Emptines and Dependent-Arising	English
15.	The Four Noble Truths	English

MINOR WORKS

1.	Mind Flower - Story book I	Tibetan
2.	Adorning the Young Mind - Story book III	Tibetan

3. Clear Lamp - Story book — Tibetan
4. Analysis of Dharma — Tibetan
5. Analysis of the World — Tibetan
6. An Introduction to Buddhism — English
7. The Doctrine of Buddhism — English

ACKNOWLEDGEMENT

The author wishes to thank all of the people who assisted in the preparation of this work who by offering their time and energy in numerous ways serve as a fine illustration of how series of inter-related events can give rise to a successful result. Tushita Retreat Centre, Dharamsala, provided the setting and was responsible for the request that the teachings be given. Effie Hanchett and Sam Doharty undertook the task of recording the teachings which were translated by Sherab Gyatso. Effie took upon herself the work of transcribing and then Tenzin Losel assiduously edited the bulk of the material, assisted in later stages by L. Chophel Gangchenpa. Effie, Ngawang Palden, Gareth Sparham and Tenzin Tsepag shared the word-processing work.